Pediatric Rheumatology in Clinical Practice

Books must be returned/renewed by the last date shown

Pediatric Rheumatology in Clinical Practice

Patricia Woo, Ronald M. Laxer, and David D. Sherry

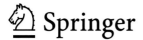 Springer

Patricia Woo, CBE, MBBS, PhD, FRCP, FMedSci
Professor of Paediatric Rheumatology, Director of the Centre for
    Paediatric and Adolescent Rheumatology, University College London
Great Ormond Street Hospital for Sick Children and University College
    Hospital, London, UK

Ronald M. Laxer, MD, FRCPC
Vice President, Clinical and Academic Affairs, The Hospital for
    Sick Children
Professor of Pediatrics and Medicine, University of Toronto, Toronto,
    Ontario, Canada

David D. Sherry, MD
Director, Clinical Rheumatology, Attending, Pain Management,
    Departments of Rheumatology and Anesthesiology, The Children's
    Hospital of Philadelphia
Professor of Pediatrics, University of Pennsylvania, Philadelphia,
    Pennsylvania, USA

British Library Cataloguing in Publication Data
A catalogue record for this book is available from the British Library

Library of Congress Control Number: 2006923490

ISBN-10: 1-84628-420-1   e-ISBN-10: 1-84628-421-X
ISBN-13: 978-1-84628-420-5   e-ISBN-13: 978-1-84628-421-2

Printed on acid-free paper

9 8 7 6 5 4 3 2 1

Springer Science+Business Media
springer.com

WS 270

A 080480

Preface

Pediatric rheumatology is a relatively new speciality, with many fascinating conditions peculiar to young people. Many of these disorders are only rarely encountered by the generalist and so often present as diagnostic dilemmas. Our aim in producing this manual is to provide easily accessible and practical information in a pocket book. We aim to assist the pediatrician, the general practitioner, as well as rheumatologists with an interest in pediatric rheumatology, in the diagnosis and management of these diseases and problems. The emphasis has been placed on clinical presentation and how to arrive at a diagnosis, and an up-to-date management plan. Brief background information on the etiology is also provided. We sincerely hope that the information herein will help decrease the impact of these conditions on the children and their families by timely diagnosis and early intervention.

Patricia Woo
Ronald M. Laxer
David D. Sherry

Contents

Preface   v

Part I Introduction   1

1. General Presentation of Musculoskeletal Problems
   in Childhood   3

2. General Principles of Management   16

**Part II Inflammatory Rheumatologic
Diseases**   21

3. Juvenile Idiopathic Arthritis (JIA)   23

4. Systemic Lupus Erythematosus (SLE)   47

5. Juvenile Dermatomyositis   66

6. Scleroderma   77

7. Overlap Syndromes   90

8. Vasculitis   97

9. Lyme Arthritis   118

10. Autoinflammatory Syndromes   123

11. Acute Rheumatic Fever and Post Streptococcal
    Arthritis   137

Part III Noninflammatory Rheumatologic Diseases 143

12. Noninflammatory Mechanical Pain Syndromes 145

13. Amplified Musculoskeletal Pain 155

14. Hereditary Conditions of Bone and Cartilage 166

Index 175

Part I

Introduction

Chapter 1
General Presentation of Musculoskeletal Problems in Childhood

1.1 INTRODUCTION

The rheumatic diseases in children range from affecting a very isolated part of the body to including almost every organ and body system. The key to making a diagnosis usually rests in the patient's history and physical examination. Paramount is the knowledge of what normal is, especially in the musculoskeletal examination. It is then, just a matter of recognizing the patterns of the various rheumatic diseases. Laboratory and imaging studies help substantiate a diagnosis, and at times are essential, so determining the most efficacious use of these resources is vital. However, there exist children who defy our classification systems and will have features of several concurrent rheumatic diseases (overlap syndromes) or just part of a disease. It may take years before enough manifestations of their disease develop before a diagnosis can be definitively made (if ever). Additionally, some children will evolve from one diagnostic category into another so one needs to always be vigilant when caring for children with rheumatic illnesses.

1.2 RHEUMATOLOGIC HISTORY

A typical rheumatologic history is on Table 1.1. Determining if a condition is inflammatory is generally the first step. Inflammation is characterised by pain, warmth, redness, swelling, and limitation of function. Some inflammatory conditions only have one or two of these findings, and 25% of children with oligoarthritis report no pain. Morning stiffness and gelling (stiffness after being still such as in a car ride) are important indicators of inflammation. However, pain and loss of function is frequent in those without inflammation so the entire picture needs to be considered before arriving at a conclusion.

1.3 FAMILY HISTORY

Many of the rheumatic diseases have a genetic basis so family history takes on an increased importance, including ethnic

TABLE 1.1. Rheumatologic History

Present Illness
  Chief complaint? (could be pain, fever, rash, fatigue, dry mouth, or other rheumatic symptoms)
  Present medications and treatments?
  Recent past medications and treatments? (for this condition and for other conditions)
  Location of pain?
  Details of onset: Acute, gradual, traumatic?
  Duration of pain?
  Severity of pain: Getting better or worse?
  Quality of pain: Stabbing, burning, freezing, aching, spasms, crushing?
  Particular time of day that it is worse or better?
  Specifically, morning, evening, or nocturnal pain?
  Does it radiate, migrate, or is it episodic?
  It is hot or cold to the touch?
  Does it look different or swollen?
  Does it interfere with functioning? School attendance, chores, recreation, activities of daily living (dressing, eating, bathing, toileting)?
  Does anything make it better or worse? Medications, rubbing, ice, heat, activity, rest, distraction?
  Between 0 and 10, how much does it hurt? (or other pain scale such as Faces Scale). Right now, highest and lowest in the past week?
  Associated symptoms? Fever, rash, weight change, weakness, sleep disturbance, depression, anxiety, behavior change, cough, vision or hearing changes, headache, abdominal pain, diarrhea, dizziness, unable to concentrate?

Past History
  Allergies
  Similar problem in the past?
  Immunization history, especially measles and hepatitis B
  Hospitalisations and surgeries
  Recent eye examination?

Social History
  Any new life events? Divorce, moving, school changes, family member changes?
  Any change in grade in school and school performance?
  Living with whom?
  Travel outside the area? Where? Tick bite? Diarrhea?

Family History
  Family members with rheumatic disease (SLE, arthritis, IBD, reactive arthritis, ankylosing spondylitis), psoriasis, back pain or spasms, even if family members know why they have back pain, heel spurs or heel pain, iritis, fibromyalgia, tuberculosis

TABLE 1.1. *Continued*

Family friends with chronic pain or infections such as tuberculosis
Family member with early stroke or heart attack, deep vein
  thrombosis or miscarriage?
Review of Systems
  Complete review needs to be taken, but specific to the rheumatic
    diseases include dry mouth or eyes, hair coming out, trouble
    swallowing, hoarse voice, frequent infections, genital sores or
    discharge, fingers turning colors in the cold, easy bruising,
    hearing changes, conjunctivitis, eye pain, vision changes,
    rashes, photosensitivity, allodynia, and weight loss

extraction, since many conditions are more frequent in select groups. One of the more common subtle clues is lower back pain that goes unreported because it is presumed to be due to trauma. Many parents with spondyloarthropathy have been diagnosed because the child presents with enthesitis related arthritis.

I.4 SOCIAL HISTORY
Social history is important especially in children with amplified musculoskeletal pain and those with chronic conditions, which will impact on the family and social functioning of the child. There is an emotional impact of all illnesses on the entire family, especially those that are chronic, life threatening, or disabling.

I.5 PAST HISTORY
Past history may reveal that the problem at hand is a recurrent problem, or is a consequence of a prior event or travel to an endemic area.

The rheumatic diseases can affect a person wherever there is a blood vessel or where there isn't, so a complete examination is mandatory. Special rheumatic investigations include a careful examination of the skin (including nails, nail fold capillaries, hair), eyes (cornea, iritis, retina), ears (hearing), all mucous membranes, teeth (apical caries), lymph nodes (epitrochlear, axillary, and supraclavicular if tumor is suspected), vessels (pulses and bruits), testes, heart (murmurs and rubs), lungs (dullness, rubs), abdomen (peritonism, tenderness, ascites, enlarged organs), nervous system (muscle tone, bulk, strength, reflexes, cranial nerves, mental states, cerebral function, sensation), and, of course, the joints, tendons, bursa and entheses. This is in addition to observing the child and family emotional interactions that may influence the child's care and diagnosis.

1.6 JOINT EXAMINATION

The joint examination is probably the hardest part to master and even seasoned rheumatologists will differ in their assessment of which joints are actively inflamed. Careful attention should be given to each joint and each joint should be felt for swelling or warmth. Rapid joint movement will elicit guarding, an early sign of inflammation. Special mention should be made about several finer points of the joint examination. The temporomandibular joint (TMJ) can be destroyed painlessly, so close attention should be given to the jaw excursion and any deviation investigated (Figure 1.1a–d). The tooth-to-tooth gap should be at least the width of the child's index, middle, and ring fingers held together (Figure 1.2). Have the child look up in order to observe for asymmetrical jaw growth. The first range to be limited in cervical spine disease is extension (check by having the child squeeze your finger between the base of their neck and occiput). Elbows are best felt by holding the arm from the medial side and palpating just lateral to the olecranon as you extend the elbow (Figure 1.3). Lower back

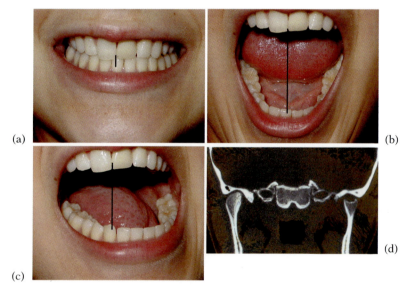

(a)

(b)

(c)

(d)

FIGURE 1.1. Normal and abnormal temporomandibular joint excursion (or jaw gait): The gap between the upper two central incisors should be compared to the lower teeth with the mouth closed (a) and remain in the relative same horizontal plane with the mouth open (b). Note that in (c) the jaw deviates to the child's right. Computerized tomography shows destruction of the right temporomandibular joint (d).

FIGURE 1.2. A quick way to check for adequate temporomandibular joint excursion: The patient should be able to get his or her own three fingers into the mouth.

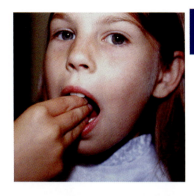

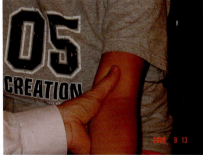

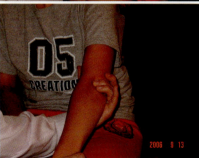

FIGURE 1.3. Proper position of the hand to examine the elbow: An effusion would be felt under the middle finger of the examiner's hand when the elbow is extended.

range of motion is ascertained by the modified Schober test. This is done by making a mark on the spine at the level of the dimples of Venus (posterior superior iliac spine) and marks 10 cm cephaled and 5 cm caudad to this mark while the patient is standing (Figure 1.4). The resulting 15 cm segment is measured when the patient leans forward and should expand to 21 cm or more. The entheses, where tendons attach to bone, need to be palpated directly, especially those shown in Figure 1.5.

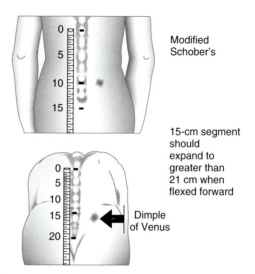

FIGURE 1.4. Modified Schober test: A mark 10 above and 5 cm below the level of the dimples of Venus should expand to 21 cm or more.

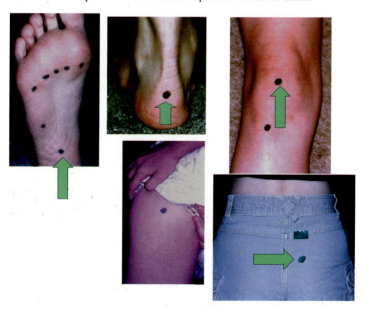

FIGURE 1.5. The enthesis is where tendons attach to bone. The sites that are the most commonly involved entheses in enthesitis-related arthritis are shown with arrows.

1.7 LABORATORY AND IMAGING STUDIES

Laboratory and imaging studies will be discussed with each clinic entity, but there are some general rules. Do not order what you do not want back. This is especially true regarding an anti-nuclear antibody (ANA) test in a child without arthritis or in whom you do not suspect lupus; up to 15% of normal children have a positive ANA test. Subsequent evaluation leads to unnecessary cost and angst. Another example is a very high alkaline phosphatase due to benign transient hyperphosphatasemia, which is common in young normal children, but also occurs in older children and even adults. One abnormal test usually does not confirm a diagnosis. Most criteria require repeated abnormalities separated by minimal periods of time such as Rheumatoid Factor (RF) in Juvenile Idiopathic Arthritis (JIA) and low blood counts in Systemic Lupus Erythematosus (SLE). The most important tests should be confirmed over time. Tests can be altered by treatment, either falsely such as urine protein tests by tolmetin, or as a function of the test such as an increase erythrocyte sedimentation rate (ESR) after administration of intravenous immunoglobulin (IVIG). Imaging is never as good as histology and shadows generated by all imaging techniques can be false or misinterpreted.

The patterns of illness can be divided into systemic and localized, and each of these can be chronic or acute (Table 1.2). Usually it is not too difficult to tell the difference, but within each of these broad areas there are subtle differences between the illnesses.

1.8 CLUES TO THE DIAGNOSIS

There are clues to the diagnosis (Table 1.3) such as JIA is almost never associated with a red joint. Keeping these points in mind will help one more quickly establish a differential diagnosis and help one select laboratory and imaging studies in a thoughtful and effective manner. We will attempt to construct algorithms in each section, but no one system is foolproof. Since there are many variations on the theme one cannot be locked into a "cookbook" approach to diagnosis or treatment and each child needs individual tailoring of diagnostic tests and therapy.

1.9 ETIOLOGY

Regarding etiology, the causes of the rheumatic diseases are unknown unless you include Lyme disease. We know the triggers for acute rheumatic fever and some for reactive arthritis, and the genes involved in most of the recurrent fever syndromes.

TABLE 1.2. Patterns of Illness

Systemic		Localized	
Acute	Chronic	Acute	Chronic
Polyarthritis	Polyarthritis	Reactive arthritis	Oligoarthritis
Acute rheumatic fever	RF+ polyarthritis JIA	Hemarthrosis	Osteoid osteoma
Kawasaki	Takayasu	Toxic synovitis	Polyarthritis
Dermatomyositis	Dermatomyositis	Lyme	Lyme
Systemic JIA	Systemic JIA	SCFE	SCFE
Septic arthritis	Diffuse pain syndromes	Localised pain syndromes	Localized pain syndromes
Malignancy	Scleroderma	Legg–Calvé–Perthes	Legg–Calvé–Perthes
SLE	SLE	Enthesitis-related arthritis	Enthesitis-related arthritis
MCTD	MCTD	Psoriatic JIA	Psoriatic JIA
Wegener granulomatosis	Wegener granulomatosis	Iridocyclitis	Iridocyclitis
Polyangiitis	Polyangiitis	Osgood–Schlatter	Osgood–Schlatter
Autoinflammatory syndromes	Autoinflammatory syndromes	PVNS	PVNS
Henoch–Schönlein purpura			Linear morphea
			Idiopathic chondrolysis
			Erythromelalgia
			Metabolic storage diseases

JIA = Juvenile Idiopathic Arthritis.
SLE = Systemic Lupus Erythematosus.
PVNS = Pigmented Villonodular Synovitis.
SCFE = Slipped Capital Femoral Epiphysis.

TABLE 1.3. Clues to Help Construct a Differential Diagnosis

Clues	Diagnoses to Consider		
Sick	Septic arthritis Osteomyelitis Acute rheumatic fever Neuroblastoma Primary vasculitis Hypertrophic pulmonary osteoarthropathy	Kawasaki Reactive arthritis Sarcoid Serum sickness Pyomyositis	Inflammatory bowel disease SLE/MCTD/JDM Leukemia Lyme Autoinflammatory syndromes Systemic JIA
Red joint	Septic arthritis Acute rheumatic fever SLE/MCTD	Osteomyelitis Reactive arthritis	Leukemia Kawasaki
Hip pain	Septic arthritis Spondyloarthropathy Toxic synovitis	Idiopathic chondrolysis Legg–Calvé–Perthes Leukemia	Osteoid osteoma Slipped epiphysis Oligoarthritis
Pain behind the knee	Benign hypermobility syndrome	Synovial cyst	BNMSPC (growing pains)
Enthesitis	Spondyloarthropathy: Ankylosing spondylitis, reactive arthritis, Inflammatory bowel disease, psoriasis, enthesopathy without arthritis	Enthesitis-related arthritis	
Enthesalgia	Aseptic necrosis: Köhler—Tarsal navicular; Kienböck—Carpel lunate; Frieberg—Second or third metatarsal head	Avulsion fracture: Osgood–Schlatter—Tibial tuberosity; Sinding-Larsen-Johansson—Patella	

TABLE 1.3. *Continued*

Clues	Diagnoses to Consider		
Dactylitis	Psoriatic arthritis	Sickle cell	Enthesitis-related arthritis
Rash	Acute rheumatic fever Dermatomyositis Kawasaki Primary vasculitis Meningococcus Autoinflammatory syndromes	Serum sickness Psoriasis Reactive arthritis Lyme Viral Systemic JIA	SLE/MCTD Inflammatory bowel disease Henoch–Schönlein purpura Gonorrhea Rocky mountain spotted fever
Not walking	*See under* Sick and monarticular pain/ arthritis, plus fracture* Discitis Systemic JIA	Osteoid osteoma Cord tumor Polyarthritis	Amplified musculoskeletal pain Myositis
Neurologic symptoms	Cerebral palsy Polyarthritis nodosa Systemic infection	Lyme Kawasaki Systemic JIA	SLE/MCTD Sarcoid Cerebral vasculitis
Clubbing	Cystic fibrosis Hypertrophic Pulmonary Osteoarthropathy	Familial	Inflammatory bowel disease
Monarticular pain/ arthritis	Septic arthritis Trauma* Osteoid osteoma Osteogenic sarcoma Oligoarthritis	Hemophilia Thorn (foreign body) Reactive Viral	Pigmented villonodular synovitis Aseptic necrosis Osteochondritis dissecans Leukemia (especially hip)

Bone pain	Leukemia Osteoid osteoma (night pain)	Fracture*	Sickle cell
Migratory arthritis	Acute rheumatic fever Palindromic rheumatism	Lyme Leukemia	Viral
Episodic arthritis	Thalassemia Palindromic rheumatism Leukemia	Sickle cell Hyperlipidemia	Familial mediterranean fever Crystal disease
Raynaud's phenomenon	Scleroderma Primary, unassociated with other diseases (can be familial)	SLE	MCTD
Allodynia	Amplified musculoskeletal pain Apprehension	Shingles	Infection
Incongruent affect	Amplified musculoskeletal pain		
Cyanosis/cold	Amplified musculoskeletal pain Arterial occlusion (APL, SLE, MCTD, Scleroderma, Vasculitis)	Raynaud's phenomenon	

*One must consider the possibility of nonaccidental injury with fractures and trauma in children.
SLE = Systemic Lupus Erythematosus.
MCTD = Mixed Connective Tissue Disease.
BNMSPC = Benign Nocturnal Musculoskeletal Pains of Childhood.
JIA = Juvenile Idiopathic Arthritis.
JDM = Juvenile Dermatomyositis.
APL = Antiphospholipid antibody syndrome.

TABLE 1.4. Number of Children with Different Rheumatic Diseases Expected in a Population of 1 Million Children*

Illness	Expected Number	Sex Predilection	Racial Predilection
Juvenile idiopathic arthritis total	2050	Overall F > M	White > Asian > Black
Oligoarticular	600	4F:1M	White
Polyarticular RF+	100	4+F:1M	White
Polyarticular RF–	400	3F:1M	White
Systemic	100	F = M	All
Psoriatic arthritis	150	F slightly > M	90% White
Enthesitis related	500	F < M	White, native American, Asian
Other	200	Probably F > M	White
Systemic lupus erythematosus	150	5–10F:1M	Black, Asian, Hispanic
Juvenile dermatomyositis/polymyositis	15	3F:1M	White
Sclerodermas	15	2F:1M systemic, F = M localized	All equal
Vasculitis syndromes	100–200	Depends on diagnosis	Variable depending on diagnosis
Lyme disease	Highly variable	F = M	Limited geographically to the tick vector; rural > urban
Recurrent fevers	Variable on racial population	Depends on diagnosis	Depends on diagnosis
Acute rheumatic fever	5	F = M	Much higher in developing countries
Pain syndromes	200–400	4F:1M	Maybe higher in upper socioeconomic groups

*For many of these conditions, the numbers are estimated based on the populations of pediatric rheumatology clinics, not on formal population studies.[1-3]

1.10 PREVALENCE

The prevalence of the rheumatic illness varies between racial groups and geography and there is scant data regarding the rarer conditions.[1-3] Table 1.4 summarizes the numbers of children with various rheumatic illnesses given a population of 1 million children.

References

1. Bowyer S, Roettcher P. Pediatric rheumatology clinic populations in the United States: results of a 3 year survey. Pediatric Rheumatology Database Research Group. *J Rheumatol*. 1996;23:1968–1974.
2. Malleson PN, Fung MY, Rosenberg AM. The incidence of pediatric rheumatic diseases: results from the Canadian Pediatric Rheumatology Association Disease Registry. *J Rheumatol*. 1996;23:1981–1987.
3. Symmons DP, Jones M, Osborne J et al. Pediatric rheumatology in the United Kingdom: data from the British Pediatric Rheumatology Group National Diagnostic Register. *J Rheumatol*. 1996;23:1975–1980.

Chapter 2
General Principles of Management

2.1 INTRODUCTION

The aim of any therapy is to address the cause and/or mechanisms of the disease. This may be done using drugs and structured rehabilitation. In some cases, psychotherapy is required. It is important to recognise that disease pathology can cause alteration in behavior, especially in the very young who are unable to articulate symptoms. Chronic illness can disturb the family dynamic and the child's education and development. Therefore, a multidisciplinary approach is frequently required to restore function and fully integrate the child back into his/her family, school and peer group. The approach should be age-appropriate. Transition to adolescence and adulthood needs to be structured. Ideally, all therapeutic methods should be subject to controlled trials to establish efficacy. However, inherent in all therapy is an element of trial and error, as there are always individual variations due to each person's unique genetic and metabolic background. The physician arrives at his/her preferred option often through a Bayesian approach, maximizing the probability of success from published data, as well as from past and collective experiences.

2.2 INFLAMMATORY/AUTOIMMUNE DISEASES

This group comprises the juvenile idiopathic arthritides (JIA), the multisystem inflammatory diseases, such as systemic lupus erythematosus (SLE), Juvenile Dermatomyositis (JDM) and the vasculitides, as well as the recurrent fever syndromes, many of which have a genetic mutation identified affecting the homeostasis of the inflammatory network. Individual descriptions of these diseases and their treatment algorithms are described in more detail in this book. Clinical guidelines for some have been published, e.g., treatment of JIA in the UK[1]. Anti-inflammatory drugs that suppress the action or synthesis of mediators of inflammation, as opposed to drugs that stimulate endogenous anti-inflammatory mediators are the first options for treating

TABLE 2.1. Anti-Inflammatory/Immunomodulatory Drugs Targeting Soluble Mediators

Drug Type	Mode of Action
NSAID	Cyclo-oxygenase 1 and 2 inhibition
Steroids	Suppress inflammatory cytokine production
Methotrexate	Suppress inflammatory cytokine production, inhibits dihydrofolate reductase, inhibits lymphocyte proliferation in high doses
Anti-TNF	Blocks the action of TNF (inflammation, T and B cell signaling, and T cell proliferation)
IL-1ra	A recombinant form of the natural receptor antagonist, and blocks cellular signaling by IL-1α and β
Anti-sIL-6R	Tocilizumab: A humanised monoclonal antibody that blocks cell signaling by the complex of IL-6/IL-6R

*Infliximab and adalimumab are, respectively, recombinant chimeric and humanised antibodies to TNFα; etanercept is a recombinant form of the naturally occurring sTNFR and blocks TNFα and LT β signaling.

‡NSAID: Nonsteroidal anti-inflammatory drugs; TNF: Tumor necrosis factor; IL-1: Interleukin 1; IL-1ra: Interleukin 1receptor antagonist; IL-6: Interleukin 6; IL-6R: Interleukin 6 receptor; sIL-6R: Soluble IL-6R.

these diseases. They include the nonsteroidal anti-inflammatory drugs (NSAIDS) that inhibit cyclo-oxygenase 1 and 2, methotrexate, steroids, and the new anti-cytokine agents (anti-TNF, IL-1ra, and anti-sIL-6R) (Table 2.1). Beyond blocking inflammatory mediators, a second class of drugs is often used in parallel. These drugs are based on their ability to alter the balance of the cellular immune response, either by depleting certain populations of lymphocytes thought to be pathogenic, or by inhibiting certain cellular functions. These include drugs such as hydroxychloroquine, leflunamide, sulfasalazine, steroid, azathioprine, mycophenolate mofetil, cyclophosphamide, cyclosporine A, and biologics in clinical trials, such as B cell depletion by monoclonal antibody against B cells (anti-CD20/rituximab) (see Table 2.2). Colchicine has been used with success in recurrent fever syndromes, small vessel vasculitis, and Behçet's, and thalidomide is particularly useful for mucocutaneous Behçet's disease. Their mode of action is not entirely clear and in vitro experiments have shown cellular effects as well as suppression of proinflammatory cytokines. Finally, autologous stem cell transplant in severe

TABLE 2.2. Immunomodulatory Drugs Targeting Cells

Drug Type	Mode of Action
High-dose IV steroids	Depletes lymphocyte numbers; blocks cell signaling
Cyclophosphamide	Depletes lymphocytes, B and T cells
Cyclosporin A	Blocks transcription of T cell genes
Mycophenolate mofetil	Inhibits B and T cell proliferation
Azathioprine	Inhibits T lymphocytes
Hydroxychloroquine	Inhibits phospholipid function and binds DNA
Sulfasalazine	Unclear
Leflunamide	Unclear
Colchicine	Inhibits cytoskeletal transport
Thalidomide	Inhibits cytokine secretions and T cell proliferation
Monoclonal antibodies to B cells	Depletes pre- and mature B cell numbers (anti-CD20/rituximab)

systemic JIA and SLE have been used with some success, but this is a treatment with an associated mortality rate of around 5% in the case of JIA. It is also an experimental medical treatment that is closely monitored by an international consortium. Specific treatment for individual diseases will be covered within the individual chapters.

2.3 PAIN IN INFLAMMATORY DISEASES

The pain threshold is lowered in children with JIA[2] and, clinically, one can encounter pain amplification in these children. The release of prostanoids and the proinflammatory cytokine IL-1 has been shown to cause pain and lower pain threshold. These mediators have direct effects on the central nervous system, in addition to their inflammatory actions peripherally. There is evidence that pain can further enhance the inflammatory response. Therefore, the management of the child should include analgesic, as well as anti-inflammatory, therapy. Physiotherapy to improve joint and muscle function may have a direct analgesic benefit. Cognitive behavioral therapy also can decrease pain and improve function.

2.4 MULTIDISCIPLINARY APPROACH TO MANAGEMENT

Inflammation causes weakening and wasting of muscle directly through the inflammatory cytokines, as well as through reflex inhibition from joint swelling and pain. In juvenile dermatomyositis, there is, additionally, inflammation of the skeletal muscles. Joint contractures frequently result. In Scleroderma, fibrosis of skin and soft tissues can cause disabling contractures without the synovium being affected. Bone development is affected by inflammation and osteoporosis can occur locally, as well as globally. The biomechanics of complex joints, such as the knee, are particularly easily deranged. Thus, specialist physiotherapy is critical during the inflammatory and rehabilitation phases. These problems are distinct from musculoskeletal rehabilitation after injury or operation, therefore the rehabilitation program for inflammatory diseases has to be different.

Pain amplification is seen in both inflammatory and noninflammatory problems and requires a multidisciplinary approach. The restoration of function is an overlap area between the physiotherapist, the podiatrist, and the occupational therapist. The latter takes a more functional approach to the child's ability to cope in the home, school and local community. Clinical and educational psychologists help with the evaluation and treatment of family dynamics and school reentry issues. Social workers help obtain necessary community and governmental (or insurance company) support.

2.5 COMPLEMENTARY AND ALTERNATIVE THERAPIES

The multidisciplinary approach to address all the needs of the child with a rheumatological problem has already been stressed. Complementary therapies, although few formal trials have been conducted, are useful for individual children[3,4]. Relaxation techniques, massage, aromatherapy and acupuncture are to control pain and should not be discouraged.

Homeopathy is a frequently used remedy. Since the remedies consist of extremely diluted substances, often diluted beyond Avogadro's number, they generally have no untoward effects.

There has been an explosion of public interest in oriental and folk remedies. Certain traditional medications from China and India have active principles similar to the drugs used in the western world, but have not undergone controlled trials. Uninformed use may lead to significant side effects, such as heavy metal nephropathy, bone marrow suppression from alkaloids, and a host of steroid side effects[5]. Some may be helpful as in the fish oils. Glucosamine and chondroitin are not anti-inflammatory but are useful in osteoarthritis in adults.

Only in cases when the practitioner of alternative medicine claims that these remedies should replace conventional drugs, in the presence of continuing clinical and laboratory signs of inflammation, should there be a clear line drawn in favor of drugs which have been demonstrated to be effective in controlled studies.

References
1. Hull RG. British Paediatric Rheumatology Group guidelines for management of childhood arthritis. *Rheumatology (Oxford)*. 2001; 40:1309–1312.
2. Hogeweg JA, Kuis W, Huygen AC et al. The pain threshold in juvenile chronic arthritis. *Br J Rheumatol*. 1995;34:61–67.
3. Shaw D, Leon C, Murray V et al. Patients' use of complementary medicine. *Lancet*. 1998;352:408.
4. Feldman DE, Duffy C, De Civita M et al. Factors associated with the use of complementary and alternative medicine in juvenile idiopathic arthritis. *Arthritis Rheum*. 2004;51:527–532.
5. Shaw D, Leon C, Kolev S et al. Traditional remedies and food supplements. A 5-year toxicological study (1991–1995). *Drug Saf*. 1997; 17:342–356.

Part II

Inflammatory Rheumatologic Diseases

Chapter 3
Juvenile Idiopathic Arthritis (JIA)

3.1 INTRODUCTION

The majority of children with rheumatologic conditions have some form of arthritis. The different categories are determined by articular and extra-articular manifestations and it may be months before one is sure of the diagnosis. Not knowing the category does not preclude treatment, but one should always be willing to change the diagnosis as the illness progresses. Juvenile idiopathic arthritis (JIA) is an umbrella term for a group of persistent arthritides lasting more than six weeks with unknown etiology (Table 3.1).[1] The pathogenesis of these diseases involves both autoimmune and genetic factors in varying combinations. Dysregulation of the immune and inflammatory systems are observed and include increased immune complexes, complement activation and disordered T_H1 and T_H2 cell interactions with predominance of T_H1 cells in the synovium. Additionally, hormonal, infectious and other environmental agents, yet to be identified, are probably involved. The term "Juvenile" refers to the onset of arthritis at 16 years of age or younger. However, it is an arbitrary distinction and, as far as we know, there are no biological reasons why these conditions cannot occur in adults. In fact, several are more common in adults, such as RF positive polyarthritis and psoriatic arthritis. Conversely, the onset of systemic and oligoarticular JIA in Caucasians is most commonly below the age of six and is rarely seen in adults.

3.2 OLIGOARTHRITIS

3.2.1 Definition

Arthritis in this group affects four or fewer joints in the first six months of disease. If more than four joints become involved after six months, it is defined as extended oligoarthritis, otherwise it is known as persistent oligoarthritis.[1]

TABLE 3.1. Juvenile Idiopathic Arthritis

Oligoarticular
  Persistent
  Extended

Polyarticular rheumatoid factor negative
Polyarticular rheumatoid factor positive
Systemic
Enthesitis-related arthritis
Psoriatic arthritis
Unclassified arthritis

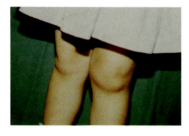

FIGURE 3.1. Unilateral arthritis of the right knee in oligoarticular JIA.

3.2.2 Epidemiology

This is the most common form of JIA and preferentially afflicts 1 to 3-year-old white girls. Although all races can be affected, the prevalence is much reduced in noncaucasians. Girls outnumber boys 4:1. It affects about 60 per 100,000 children.

3.2.3 Etiology

About 70% of oligoarticular JIA patients have antinuclear antibodies and there is a disproportionate number with the HLA alleles at DR8 (DRB1*0801) and DR5 (DRB1*1104) loci.[2] Other factors may be at play, giving rise to the predominance of girls.

3.2.4 Clinical Manifestations

Approximately half of oligoarticular JIA patients will have a single joint involved at onset, mainly the knee (Figure 3.1). The next most commonly affected joint is the ankle (Figure 3.2). Small joints of the hand are the third most commonly affected, but it may portend the later onset of psoriatic arthritis.[3] Temporomandibular Joint (TMJ) arthritis is not uncommon, but is often detected late in the course of the disease, as symptoms are not common. Initial wrist involvement is rare and may indicate the progression to extended oligoarthritis, or polyarticular disease. Shoulders are almost never involved. Cervical spine

FIGURE 3.2. Posterior view of unilateral arthritis of the left ankle, showing valgus deformity of the hind foot.

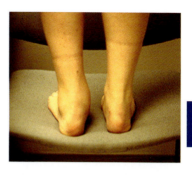

3

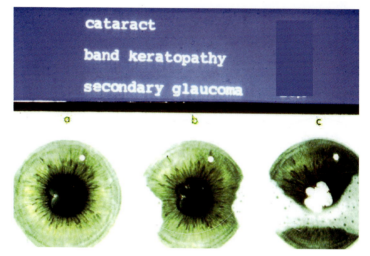

FIGURE 3.3. Complications of iridocyclitis of JIA. Left to right: Cataract, synecheae, band keratopathy. Late outcome is secondary glaucoma.

disease may be manifest by torticollis. Iridocyclitis, usually noted by an irregular pupil, is rarely a presenting sign. The anterior uveitis (iridocyclitis) is low grade and early inflammation is only detectable by slit lamp examination.

Most children will complain of pain, morning stiffness and gelling and a parent will notice a limp and joint swelling. However, 25% of children report no pain and only swelling is observed.

The most common extra-articular manifestation is iridocyclitis. In oligoarthritis up to 20% of patients can develop iridocyclitis, which is usually asymptomatic. The eye is neither red nor photophobic. It is more prevalent in the children who are ANA positive. The astute physician should look for keratopunctate deposits on the cornea or synechiae at presentation (Figure 3.3) and, if present, should send the child immediately for an ophthalmologic consultation; if absent, the child should have a slit lamp examination of the eyes every three to four months for the first year regardless. Some physicians will decrease the surveillance to every six months if the ANA is negative, since a positive ANA test is a strong predictor of iridocyclitis[4] (Table 3.2).

3.2.5 Laboratory Features

The most common abnormal finding is a low titre positive ANA test, usually 1:40 to 1:320 depending on the test system. It is present in 50–70% of children with oligoarthritis. Occasionally, the child will have elevated acute phase reactants, such as an elevated ESR or CRP, but these are usually mildly elevated. Greatly elevated acute phase reactants may be associated with subclinical Inflammatory Bowel Disease. The blood counts remain normal and the RF is negative.

3.2.6 Establishing the Diagnosis

The diagnosis is made by the presence of chronic arthritis (longer than six weeks) in four or fewer joints in the first six months of disease and the absence of other causes.

Exclusions to oligoarthritis include psoriasis in a first- or second-degree relative, HLA-B27 associated disease in a first-degree relative, systemic JIA, a positive RF test, or a positive HLA-B27 test in a boy aged six years or older. Table 3.3 is a general outline to assist in the diagnosis of children with various forms of JIA.

The differential diagnosis is broadest in monoarticular arthritis and includes septic arthritis, reactive arthritis, foreign body synovitis, pigmented villonodular synovitis, arterial-venous malformation, bleeding disorders (such as hemophilia), or severe trauma, including non-accidental trauma (Table 1.3). Routine trauma, such as from a fall, does not cause persistent joint swelling and trauma is very rarely a cause of joint swelling unless there is an internal derangement seen in older, not younger, children. Lyme disease (in an endemic area) frequently causes knee swelling usually for less than six weeks, although it is frequently recurrent. Leukemia can cause limb pain and may be associated with swelling, but is associated usually with systemic manifestations and more pain and disability than in children with JIA.[5]

TABLE 3.2. Recommended Frequency of Slit Lamp Examination to Check for Asymptomatic Iridocyclitis for Children with JIA

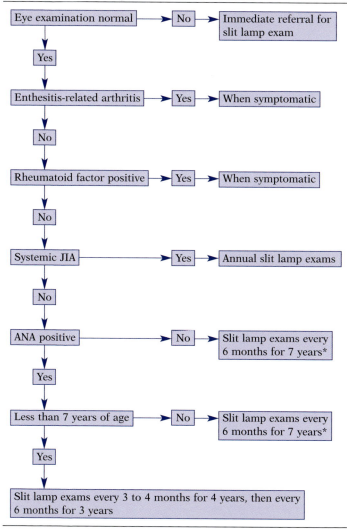

*Some physicians will have these children get a slit lamp examination every 3 to 4 months initially for 1 to 2 years since it is possible for ANA-negative children to develop iridocyclitis. Usually, after 7 years, exams can be annual. If iridocyclitis develops, then this scheme does not apply, and the frequency of slit lamp exams will be more frequent as per the ophthalmologist.

TABLE 3.3. Algorithm for the Diagnosis of JIA*

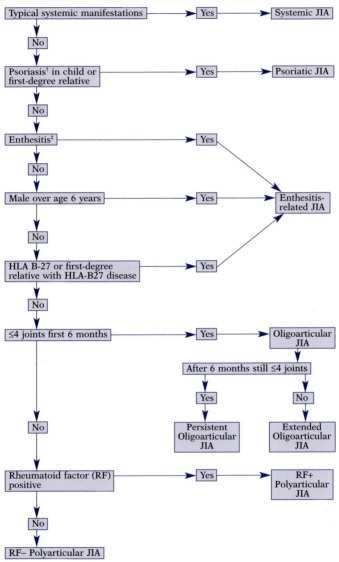

---

* These are general guidelines, since there are specific exclusions not fully outlined. A few children will qualify as having either none or two forms of JIA and are, therefore, classified as having Unclassified JIA. The arthritis is defined in the ILAR classification as occurring in a child of 16 or under, and persisting for over 6 weeks.
† Psoriasis confirmed by a physician.
‡ Number and site of tender entheses not specified; we prefer at least 3 sites other than metatarsal heads.

3.2.7 Treatment

The initial treatment should be intra-articular injection with tri-amcinolone hexacetonide, 1 mg/kg in knee joints and young people should be sedated. This treatment is expected to last approximately one year[6] (Table 3.4). NSAIDs may help control symptoms, but they do not alter the natural history. If the arthritis recurs, joint injections can be repeated up to three times in a 12-month period. The response to a second joint injection is not predicted by the response of the first. However, if it is resistant to multiple injections, then a disease-modifying agent, such as methotrexate, sulfasalazine, or an anti-TNF agent should be used, especially if extended disease has developed. Some physicians would add a disease modifying agent at the time of an injection of a hip or the temporomandibular joint, since these are particularly prone to destruction. In addition, they are important for function and are hard to evaluate clinically once disease has been established. Rarely, synovectomy will be required.

A few children will have persistent flexion contractures that will require physiotherapy. Besides exercise and stretching, night splints and serial casting may be required. Serial casting is done two or three times a week for up to a month if needed. Some children with marked leg length discrepancy (resulting from overgrowth of the affected knee) may require a shoe lift/raise. Iridocyclitis is usually controlled with topical medications, but if it is resistant or side effects develop, methotrexate has been shown to help.[7] Cyclosporine, tacrolimus, or infliximab may have a role should methotrexate fail.

3.2.8 Outcome

Most children with oligoarthritis do well and the disease will remit in as many as 65% over the years for the persistent oligoarthritic subgroup.[8,9] In about 20–30% of these children oligoarthritis becomes extended and the outcome is poor until methotrexate is introduced as the treatment of choice. Remission is induced in 60–70% while on methotrexate. Anti-TNF agents are effective if patients fail to respond fully to methotrexate, especially if given in combination with methotrexate. The worst outcome is visual loss, which is more frequent in children with significant eye involvement at the time of their first ophthalmologic visit. Other sequelae include leg length discrepancy, especially in those with knee arthritis. Persistent swelling and pain also lead to muscle atrophy. Thigh atrophy in children with knee arthritis is often permanent.

TABLE 3.4. Algorithm of a Way to Treat Persistent Oligoarticular JIA and Psoriatic JIA*

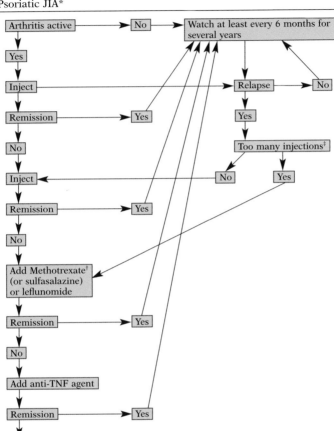

* NSAIDs are used for symptomatic care, such as morning stiffness or musculoskeletal pain. They are withdrawn once remission is achieved. Physical and occupational therapies are used as needed.
† Methotrexate and subsequent agent, if needed, are added at the time of first injection of the hip or temporomandibular joint, due to the inaccessibility of monitoring recurrent arthritis. Midfoot arthritis may also be an indication for more early addition of methotrexate and subsequent agents.
‡ The number of acceptable total injections and injections per year has not been strictly defined and will vary depending on the patient, joint, and physician. If a single joint requires more than 3 injections in a 12-month period, many rheumatologists would add a DMARD.

3.3 POLYARTHRITIS, RHEUMATOID FACTOR (RF) NEGATIVE

3.3.1 Definition
Arthritis affecting five or more joints in the first six months of the disease and a negative RF test.[1]

3.3.2 Epidemiology
This form of JIA also preferentially afflicts 1 to 3 year old white girls, although all races can be affected. Girls outnumber boys 3:1. It affects about 40 per 100,000 children.

3.3.3 Etiology
Unknown, but about 40% have antinuclear antibodies.

3.3.4 Clinical Manifestations
The arthritis is usually insidious and symmetrical, frequently involving the small joints, including the distal interphalangeal joints. The children with less than 10 arthritic joints are frequently more like those with oligoarthritis than those with widespread arthritis. Iridocyclitis occurs in 5%, generally those with relatively few affected joints.

3.3.5 Laboratory Features
Polyarthritis may be associated with elevated acute phase reactants and mild anemia. The ANA test is positive in up to 40% and the RF is negative by definition.

3.3.6 Establishing the Diagnosis
The diagnosis requires arthritis to be present in five or more joints for at least six weeks. The RF test has to be negative (Table 3.3). Other major diagnostic considerations include autoimmune connective tissue diseases (particularly in the older girl who is ANA positive), lymphoma, leukaemia, or prolonged viral synovitis.

3.3.7 Treatment
Children with polyarthritis generally require a disease-modifying agent at the time of diagnosis, or shortly after the diagnosis is firmly established (Table 3.5). If, within several months (maximum six) methotrexate is not working well enough, or is not tolerated, an anti-TNF agent (etanercept, infliximab, or adalimumab) is indicated.[10] Both reduce the progression of erosive disease. Furthermore, the combination of methotrexate and etanercept has recently been shown to be the only combination that prevents bony erosion in adults with RA. The use of

TABLE 3.5. Algorithm of a Way to Treat Extended Oligoarticular JIA and Polyarticular JIA, both RF Negative and RF Positive, with disease-modifying agents

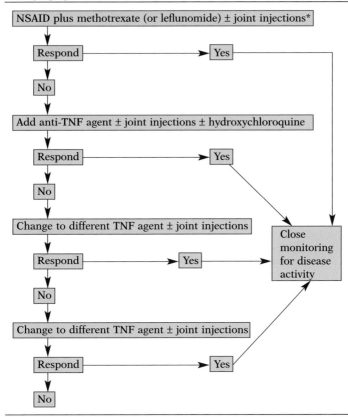

*NSAIDs are used for symptomatic care, such as morning stiffness or musculoskeletal pain. They are withdrawn once remission is achieved. Temporomandibular joint and hip arthritis should be injected early on, due to the importance of these joints to function. Physical and occupational therapies are used as needed.

sulfasalazine and leflunomide are also options before starting an anti-TNF agent in mild disease. Some children require multiple joint injections to maintain control of the arthritis and function, as well as physical and occupational therapy.

3.3.8 Outcome
Approximately 50% (or less) of children will go into long-term remission, but usually only after years.[11] As a result, there are

often significant physical and psychological sequelae. Children without hip and shoulder arthritis do better and rarely become significantly disabled.

3.4 POLYARTHRITIS, RHEUMATOID FACTOR (RF) POSITIVE

3.4.1 Definition
Arthritis which affects 5 or more joints in the first 6 months of disease and a positive RF tests on 2 occasions at least 3 months apart.

3.4.2 Epidemiology
This form of JIA is more typically seen in adolescent girls. It affects about 10 per 100,000 children.

3.4.3 Etiology
Unknown, but it is associated with HLA-DR4, as in adult rheumatoid arthritis.

3.4.4 Clinical Manifestations
The arthritis is usually insidious and symmetrical, frequently involving the small joints of the hands, typically the PIP joints and wrists, with initial sparing of the MCPs. These children frequently have more than 30 joints with arthritis. At onset low-grade fever may be present, but it is distinctly different from systemic JIA. Felty syndrome (splenomegaly and leukopenia) can occur in childhood RF+ polyarthritis. Iridocyclitis is not a feature of this onset type.

3.4.5 Laboratory Features
Polyarthritis may be associated with elevated acute phase reactants and anemia. The ANA test is positive in a few and the RF is positive on two occasions three months apart. Rheumatoid factor is an IgM-anti-IgG. In these patients, anti-cyclic citrullinated peptide antibodies (anti-CCP) may be more specific and portend destructive arthritis.[12]

3.4.6 Establishing the Diagnosis
The diagnosis requires arthritis to be present in five or more joints for at least six weeks. The RF test has to be positive on two different occasions three months apart (Table 3.3). Most other diagnostic considerations are eliminated by the time the RF test is repeated and positive again.

3.4.7 Treatment

Children with RF positive polyarthritis are at high risk for prolonged erosive arthritis and will require a disease-modifying agent at the time of diagnoses (Table 3.5). Anti-TNF agents should be added if methotrexate is not adequately controlling the arthritis, since they have been shown to prevent bony erosions, especially in combination with methotrexate. Some children require multiple joint injections to maintain control of the arthritis and function and usually require physical and occupational therapy.

3.4.8 Outcome

Children with RF positive polyarthritis have long lasting disease that will require continued medication for decades. If controlled, the functional outcome can be quite good. However, there are children who do not respond and will have joint deformity and permanent dysfunction.

3.5 SYSTEMIC JIA (sJIA)

3.5.1 Definition

Arthritis with quotidian spiking fevers of ≥39 degrees Celsius for more than two weeks, accompanied by at least one of the following: an evanescent rash, lymphadenopathy, serositis, or hepatosplenomegaly. Rheumatoid factor test is negative.

3.5.2 Epidemiology

This occurs in young children with a peak age of onset between 18 months and two years in one cohort in London, UK. The median age, in most series, is around four years of age. The incidence is the same in both sexes in Caucasians, unlike the other types of JIA. The prevalence of sJIA approximates to 10 cases per 100,000, although some surveys have suggested that it may be more frequent in Japan and India.

3.5.3 Etiology

There is no association between HLA and sJIA in Caucasians. However, there is evidence that genetic predisposition comprises at least part of the cause for developing sJIA. Non-HLA genes, such as macrophage migration inhibitory factor (MIF) and Interferon Regulatory Factor (IRF), have been shown to be associated with JIA as a whole and a variant of the interleukin-6 (IL-6) gene confers susceptibility.[13] These genes predispose the patient to a vigorous inflammatory response to stimuli, such as infectious agents, and the net effect of the interaction between pro and anti-inflammatory proteins is probably the key to the clinical features in this subtype of JIA.

3.5.4 Clinical Manifestations

The fever is typically spiking in character with a peak of at least 39°C (Figure 3.4). It occurs once or twice a day and recurs each day. This is accompanied by an evanescent salmon pink macular/urticarial rash (Figure 3.5). The macular rash can be itchy. The child is usually unwell and irritable during the fever, but often recovers in between. Other accompanying symp-

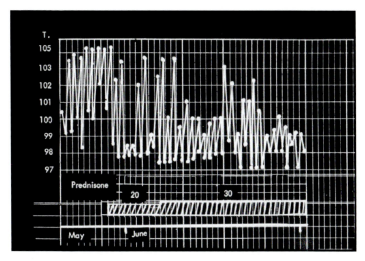

FIGURE 3.4. Daily spiking fever of systemic JIA, despite high-dose prednisolone (>2 mg/kg) in a 5-year-old.

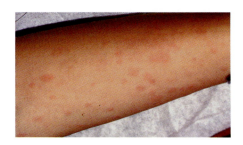

FIGURE 3.5. Typical rash of systemic JIA, which is centripetal in distribution and evanescent.

toms are headaches (sometimes with signs of meningism), arthralgia or arthritis, myalgia, abdominal pains from serositis that can mimic an acute abdomen, breathlessness and chest pains on lying flat indicating pericarditis, as well as acute chest pains from pleuritis. There is a wide variation in the severity of symptoms, ranging from fever and rash for two to three weeks followed by mild arthritis, to simultaneous onset of all the symptoms described above. In the most severe cases, they may also present with features of secondary hemophagocytic lymphohistiocytosis (HLH, also known as macrophage activation syndrome), with signs of anemia, jaundice and purpura in the later stages.[14]

3.5.5 Laboratory Features
There are no specific tests for sJIA, but there are characteristic patterns of laboratory abnormalities. There is typically a very high CRP, ESR, neutrophilia, thrombocytosis and anemia, which may be profound. Liver enzymes and coagulation screen may be abnormal in the more severe cases and certainly in HLH. There are no autoantibodies, or rheumatoid factor and complement levels are normal or high (as acute phase reactants).

3.5.6 Establishing a Diagnosis
There are many illnesses in one to two year olds that can mimic sJIA (Table 3.6). Apart from arthritis, the fever is classic and a careful fever chart will often help eliminate some of the differential diagnoses. The rash is like a viral exanthema, but the difference is that it is evanescent. If these criteria are not fulfilled unequivocally, it is necessary to screen for infectious agents, urinary vanillomandelic acids and a bone marrow aspirate to exclude infection, neuroblastoma and leukemia respectively. Some physicians do these tests routinely, since malignancies are often close mimics in the early stages of sJIA. The recurrent fevers syndromes (see Chapter 8) are often mistaken for sJIA, but the character of the fevers and the fixed rashes associated with these syndromes should alert the clinician to a different diagnosis.

3.5.7 Treatment
Mild sJIA often needs nothing more than NSAIDs given to cover the whole 24-hour period. Indomethacin is particular helpful for fever and pericarditis. Intravenous immunoglobulins are sometimes used with effect in the milder systemics when given at onset and in the mild relapsing systemic variety (see "outcome"

TABLE 3.6. Differential Diagnoses of Systematic JIA (sJIA)

Condition	Differentiating Features from sJIA
Infections	Positive cultures/antibodies, continuous fever and rash
Leukemia	Nonquotidian fevers, bone pain, systemically unwell constantly
Neuroblastoma	Nonquotidian fevers, systemically unwell constantly
CINCA/NOMID	Fixed rash, undulating fevers, neurologic complications
Kawasaki disease	Fixed rash, mucocutaneous symptoms, coronary artery dilatation
Other primary vasculitis	Undulating fevers, fixed and painful rashes or purpura, systemically ill constantly, renal involvement
SLE	Constant fevers, positive ANA and dsDNA, cytopenias, other organs involved

CINCA: Chronic infantile neurologic cutaneous and articular syndrome; NOMID: Neonatal onset multisystem inflammatory disease; SLE: Systemic lupus erythematosus.

below). In the more severe cases, steroids are needed, as well as other disease modifying drugs, such as methotrexate and cyclosporine A. There is evidence that these are less effective than in polyarthritis and some DMARDs are associated with HLH in patients with sJIA (e.g., sulphasalazine, gold, azathioprine and methotrexate), although HLH can arise in untreated children with sJIA as well. HLH in sJIA is usually effectively treated with cyclosporine A accompanied by parenteral steroids. Etanercept is less effective in sJIA as compared to polyarthritis. Newer biologics to block IL-6 and IL-1 signalling are more promising, but phase II/III trials need to be done. Table 3.7 is an algorithm of a method of treatment of sJIA.

3.5.8 Outcome
sJIA is heterogeneous in severity, disease course and outcome. It can be monocyclic, with remission within two to four years. It can relapse and be characterized by flares of systemic features with mild arthritis. Or it can continue with persistent destructive arthritis, which is usually more prominent after the regression of systemic features. Patients with severe disease can have flares

TABLE 3.7. Algorithm of a Way to Treat Systemic JIA

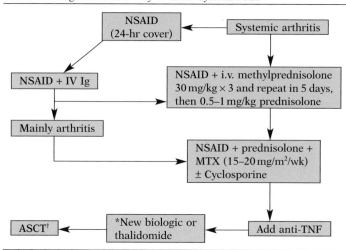

*Anakinra and anti-IL-6 receptor have been reported to be effective.
†ASCT: Autologous stem cell transplant; MTX: Methotrexate; Ig: Immunoglobulin.

of extra-articular features at any time, and 23 to 30% from two large European series had systemic features 10 to 15 years after onset.[15] Patients at the severe end of the disease spectrum usually have active arthritis into adult life despite standard therapies. Predictors of poor outcome include the presence of systemic features six months after onset, thrombocytosis and the presence of polyarthritis with hip involvement.[16] A recent review of all retrospective outcome studies, which includes psychological and functional outcomes, suggests that no clear outcome figures can be derived, partly due to the size and lack of homogeneity of the cohorts, as well as the lack of consensus on methodology. Long-term prospective studies are in progress.

The incidence of amyloidosis and surgical intervention, such as hip replacements, was much higher in the systemic subtype of JIA, and death from amyloidosis in the 1960s and 1970s used to be 50%. The mortality rate for sJIA is still perceived to be higher than the mortality rate associated with other subtypes of JIA in clinical practice now, although no formal figures are available. As a result of the inadequate control of the disease with the available therapies, growth failure and osteoporosis are serious and lasting complications. Social isolation and unemployment have also been described as more prevalent in this group.[17]

3.6 ENTHESITIS-RELATED ARTHRITIS (ERA)

3.6.1 Definition

Arthritis and/or enthesitis with at least two of the following: (1) sacroiliac joint tenderness, or inflammatory lumbosacral pain; (2) HLA-B27 positive; (3) first degree relative with medically confirmed HLA-B27 associated disease; (4) anterior iridocyclitis, usually symptomatic; and (5) onset of arthritis in a boy six years or older.

3.6.2 Epidemiology

This form of JIA is more frequent in boys, although it may be under-recognized in symptomatic girls who can have milder disease.[18] The onset typically occurs in children over six and there is a familial predilection. It may be as common as 50 per 100,000 children.

3.6.3 Etiology

ERA is generally thought to be a form of spondyloarthropathy and can be associated with HLA-B27. In patients who have the HLA-B27 gene, molecular mimicry is thought to play a role, especially regarding Klebsiella and arthritis following infections with Salmonella, Shigella, Campylobacter, Yersinia, Chlamydia, Mycoplasma, Clostridia, or even Giardia.

3.6.4 Clinical Manifestations

The defining feature of this condition is the presence of enthesitis. Enthesitis is inflammation of the tendons and ligaments where they attach to bone (the enthesis) (Figure 3.6). Not all entheses are equally significant in ERA and some are prone to mechanical damage, such as in Osgood–Schlatter and Sinding–Larsen–Johansson Syndrome (Chapter 12). Metatarsalgia is not uncommon in children and should not count as enthesitis. One study suggests that pathologic enthesitis be defined as the presence of 3 of 8 sites tested tender to palpation with about 3 to 4 kg of digital pressure.[19] These sites are: the SI joint, inferior pole of the patella, the Achilles tendon and plantar fascia insertions into the calcaneus. This work has not been confirmed, but it does emphasise that care needs to be taken in establishing the presence of enthesitis.

3.6.5 Laboratory Features

There is no defining laboratory test, although the presence of HLA-B27 is common and helps establish this diagnosis. Some

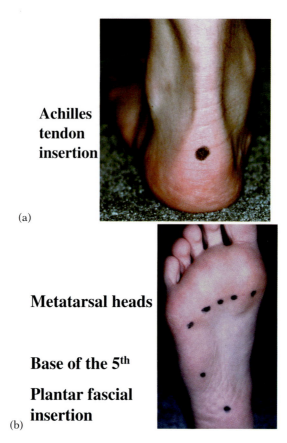

Achilles tendon insertion

(a)

Metatarsal heads

Base of the 5th

Plantar fascial insertion

(b)

FIGURE 3.6. (a) Enthesis of the Tendo Achilles, where pain is often present in enthesitis-related arthritis. (b) Entheses of the various tendon and fascial insertions of the foot: Plantar fasciitis or heel pain is a frequent symptom of enthesitis-related arthritis.

children will have a very high ESR or anemia leading to the suspicion that they may have subclinical inflammatory bowel disease. Ultrasound can distinguish enthesitis.

3.6.6 Establishing a Diagnosis

The diagnosis requires enthesitis or asymmetrical arthritis of the large joints of the lower limbs. Enthesitis or asymmetrical arthritis affects mainly preteen and teenage boys. SI joint and spinal inflammation occurs in a minority of children with ERA from about 11 years of age (Table 3.3). A classical symptom of SI joint

TABLE 3.8. Criteria for Ankylosing Spondylitis

New York Criteria

Clinical Criteria
Limitation of lumbar motion in all 3 planes
History or the presence of pain in the lumbar spine
<2.5 cm of chest excursion at the 4th intercostals space

Definite AS
Grade 3 to 4 (moderate to ankylosed) bilateral sacroiliac changes
on radiograph and at least 1 clinical criterion
Grade 3 to 4 unilateral or grade 2 (minimal) bilateral sacroiliac
changes on radiograph with criterion 1 or criteria 2 and 3

Probable AS
Grade 3 to 4 bilateral sacroiliac changes on radiograph without
clinical criteria

inflammation is buttock pain with early morning stiffness that improves with activity. Early onset of inflammatory spinal pain usually occurs in the thoracolumbar junction with stiffness and pain after rest that improves with activity. Exclusions from the diagnosis include systemic features of sJIA, a positive rheumatoid factor, psoriasis or the presence of psoriasis in a first-degree relative.

ERA overlaps with a group of conditions collectively known as spondyloarthropathies, such as Ankylosing Spondylitis (AS). AS may be heralded by enthesitis. There are several criteria for AS (Table 3.8) and young people with AS frequently, but not always, satisfy the criteria for ERA. Likewise, children who satisfy the criteria for the European Spondylarthropathy Study Group (ESSG) criteria[20] (Table 3.9) could be classified as having ERA, although psoriasis is part of the ESSG criteria and is excluded in ERA. Reactive arthritis usually occurs two to four weeks after an infection, is more frequent in children below the age of 10 and typically lasts less than six weeks. However, there are some children with prolonged reactive arthritis, or long-standing arthritis associated with inflammatory bowel disease, who have enthesitis and would be classified as having ERA until IBD is discovered.

There are few conditions that mimic ERA, although children with widespread amplified musculoskeletal pain (see Chapter 12) frequently have very tender entheses that may be mistaken for enthesitis.

TABLE 3.9. Classification Criteria of the European Spondylarthropathy Study Group (ESSG)

Inflammatory spinal pain*
Or
Synovitis (asymmetric or predominantly in the lower extremities)
Plus
One of the following:
Enthesopathy Sacroiliitis Alternating buttock pain Family history of spondylarthropathy Inflammatory bowel disease Psoriasis Urethritis, cervicitis, or diarrhea within 1 month before the onset of arthritis

*Inflammatory spinal pain is defined as pain that is worse with rest, frequently morning stiffness that improves with activity.

3.6.7 Treatment

Treatment of arthritis is similar to oligoarthritis and polyarthritis. Most patients respond to intra-articular corticosteroid injections and many will need sulfasalazine, or methotrexate, along with physiotherapy. If severe, a course of intravenous pulse methylprednisolone is often helpful. Children with enthesitis will generally require a NSAID for symptomatic relief. We empirically favour certain NSAIDs for enthesitis, specifically diclofenac, indomethacin and piroxicam. The aim of treatment is for functional relief since 100% relief is usually not attained. Occasionally corticosteroid injection of the plantar fascial insertion on the calcaneus is helpful, or for a limited time, oral steroids. Physiotherapy as well as shoe modification can help greatly.

These measures have not proved to significantly modify the course of disease, in particular, axial inflammation. The anti-TNF agents, infliximab and etanercept, have been shown to be the only effective agents for Axial Disease.[21,22] Anti-TNF agents should be used early in the course of axial disease, before irreversible damage from spinal erosion and fusion occurs. Anti-TNF agents are also associated with dramatic improvement in peripheral arthritis and enthesitis.[23]

3.6.8 Outcome

The long-term outcome is unknown. Enthesitis is more symptomatic in teens and young adults, and it improves with age. Boys
with HLA-B27 and hip arthritis, or tarsitis, are at high risk of
developing progressive spinal involvement. In Mexico, the vast
majority of boys with tarsitis later developed ankylosing
spondylitis.

3.7 PSORIATIC ARTHRITIS

3.7.1 Definition

Arthritis and psoriasis, or arthritis and at least two of the following: (1) dactylitis, (2) nail abnormalities (two or more nail
pits, or onycholysis), or (3) family history of psoriasis in a first-
degree relative.

3.7.2 Epidemiology

Psoriasis occurs in approximately 2% of the population and about
a quarter of these have arthritis. It is estimated that psoriatic
arthritis affects 15 per 100,000 children. In the United States, it is
much more common in white people than other racial groups;
approximately 90% of patients are white. Girls are slightly more
affected than boys and the typical age of onset is between 7 and
10 years, with psoriasis typically occurring within 2 years of the
onset of arthritis, although it can follow the arthritis by decades.

3.7.3 Etiology

Unknown, but there is a strong genetic component with 40% of
patients with psoriasis having a relative affected and several can-
didate genes have been identified.

3.7.4 Clinical Manifestations

The arthritis is typically asymmetric, involves both large and
small joints, and the total number of joints is limited. It is associated with asymptomatic iridocyclitis in 15% of children. These
features are typical of oligoarthritis and many children are first
classified as having oligoarticular JIA before psoriasis is manifest in the child or relative. Children with small joint involvement
of the hand tend to develop psoriatic arthritis, nearly one-third
have DIP joint involvement and up to half have dactylitis (Figure
3.7). Children with HLA-B27 develop axial disease similar to
ankylosing spondylitis. Rarely, arthritis mutilans occurs with
marked joint destruction.

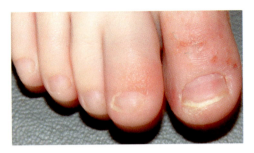

FIGURE 3.7. Dactylitis in psoriatic arthritis, with accompanying nail dystrophy.

3.7.5 Laboratory Features
The ANA test is positive in up to half of the children with psoriatic arthritis. By definition the RF is negative.

3.7.6 Establishing the Diagnosis
The diagnosis is best established when a child with chronic arthritis has psoriasis. Nail changes (i.e., multiple nail pits), dactylitis, or psoriasis in a first-degree relative are supportive (Table 3.3). Exclusions include positive rheumatoid factor, HLA-B27 disease in first-degree relatives or the child, or sJIA.

3.7.7 Treatment
The treatment is similar to oligoarthritis; intra-articular corticosteroid injections are greatly beneficial for those with limited arthritis (Table 3.4). NSAIDs help with symptoms, such as morning stiffness, but do not alter the long-term outcome.[24] Methotrexate is of great benefit for both psoriasis and arthritis and, when used in children, we recommend a single weekly dose rather than split doses more commonly used by dermatologists for psoriasis alone. In children with more aggressive disease, anti-TNF therapy is indicated and may significantly limit bony destruction. Oral corticosteroids are rarely needed.

3.7.8 Outcome
Children with psoriatic arthritis tend to have longer lasting disease, and a small but significant percentage (up to 10%) may be disabled. The iridocyclitis of psoriatic arthritis can, rarely, lead to blindness, so close monitoring is indicated (Table 3.2).

3.7.9 Unclassified Arthritis

Up to 10% of children with chronic arthritis cannot be classified by the above criteria. This is either because they do not fit a category, or they fit more than one category. Children with undifferentiated JIA are followed with a diagnosis of just chronic arthritis and may eventually become diagnosable, e.g., develop psoriasis, or enthesitis, or a connective tissue disease. Regardless of being classifiable, or not, it is always best to be flexible in our thinking about these diseases and constantly on alert for new manifestations that will change our original diagnosis.

References

1. Petty RE, Southwood TR, Manners P et al. International League of Associations for Rheumatology classification of juvenile idiopathic arthritis: second revision, Edmonton, 2001. *J Rheumatol.* 2004;31:390–392.
2. Prahalad S. Genetics of juvenile idiopathic arthritis: an update. *Curr Opin Rheumatol.* 2004;16:588–594.
3. Huemer C, Malleson PN, Cabral DA et al. Patterns of joint involvement at onset differentiate oligoarticular juvenile psoriatic arthritis from pauciarticular juvenile rheumatoid arthritis. *J Rheumatol.* 2002;29:1531–1535.
4. American Academy of Pediatrics Section on Rheumatology and Section on Ophthalmology: Guidelines for ophthalmologic examinations in children with juvenile rheumatoid arthritis. *Pediatrics.* 1993;92:295–296.
5. Trapani S, Grisolia F, Simonini G et al. Incidence of occult cancer in children presenting with musculoskeletal symptoms: a 10-year survey in a pediatric rheumatology unit. *Semin Arthritis Rheum.* 2000;29:348–359.
6. Zulian F, Martini G, Gobber D et al. Comparison of intra-articular triamcinolone hexacetonide and triamcinolone acetonide in oligoarticular juvenile idiopathic arthritis. *Rheumatology (Oxford),* 2003;42:1254–1259.
7. Foster CS. Diagnosis and treatment of juvenile idiopathic arthritis-associated uveitis. *Curr Opin Ophthalmol.* 2003;14:395–398.
8. Guillaume S, Prieur AM, Coste J et al. Long-term outcome and prognosis in oligoarticular-onset juvenile idiopathic arthritis. *Arthritis Rheum.* 2000;43:1858–1865.
9. Ravelli A, Martini A. Early predictors of outcome in juvenile idiopathic arthritis. *Clin Exp Rheumatol.* 2003;21:S89–93.
10. Horneff G, Schmeling H, Biedermann T et al. The German etanercept registry for treatment of juvenile idiopathic arthritis. *Ann Rheum Dis.* 2004;63:1638–1644.
11. Haugen M, Lien G, Flatø B et al. Young adults with juvenile arthritis in remission attain normal peak bone mass at the lumbar spine and forearm. *Arthritis Rheum.* 2000;43:1504–1510.

12. Forslind K, Ahlmen M, Eberhardt K et al. Prediction of radiological outcome in early rheumatoid arthritis in clinical practice: role of antibodies to citrullinated peptides (anti-CCP). *Ann Rheum Dis.* 2004;63:1090–1095.

13. Ogilvie EM, Fife MS, Thompson SD et al. The -174G allele of the interleukin-6 gene confers susceptibility to systemic arthritis in children: a multicenter study using simplex and multiplex juvenile idiopathic arthritis families. *Arthritis Rheum.* 2003;48:3202–3206.

14. Woo P. Systemic juvenile idiopathic arthritis: diagnosis, management and outcome. *Nat Clin Pract Rheumatol.* 2006;2:28–34.

15. Hafner R, Truckenbrodt H. Course and prognosis of systemic juvenile chronic arthritis–retrospective study of 187 patients. *Klin Padiatr.* 1986;198:401–407.

16. Spiegel LR, Schneider R, Lang BA, Birdi N, Silverman ED, Laxer RM. et al. Early predictors of poor functional outcome in systemic-onset juvenile rheumatoid arthritis: a multicenter cohort study. *Arthritis Rheum.* 2000;43:2402–2409.

17. Packham JC, Hall MA. Long-term follow-up of 246 adults with juvenile idiopathic arthritis: education and employment. *Rheumatology (Oxford),* 2002;41:1436–1439.

18. Burgos-Vargas R, Pacheco-Tena C, Vazquez-Mellado J. Juvenile-onset spondyloarthropathies. *Rheum Dis Clin North Am.* 1997;23:569–598.

19. Sherry DD, Sapp LR. Enthesalgia in childhood: site-specific tenderness in healthy subjects and in patients with seronegative enthesopathic arthropathy. *J Rheumatol.* 2003;30:1335–1340.

20. Dougados M, van der Linden S, Juhlin R, Huitfeldt B, Amor B, Calin A et al. The European Spondylarthropathy Study Group preliminary criteria for the classification of spondylarthropathy. *Arthritis Rheum.* 1991;34:1218–1227.

21. Henrickson M, Reiff A. Prolonged efficacy of etanercept in refractory enthesitis-related arthritis. *J Rheumatol.* 2004;31:2055–2061.

22. Tse SM, Burgos-Vargas R, Laxer RM. Anti-tumor necrosis factor alpha blockade in the treatment of juvenile spondylarthropathy. *Arthritis Rheum.* 2005;52:2103–2108.

23. Tse SM, Laxer RM, Babyn PS et al. Radiologic improvement of juvenile idiopathic arthritis-enthesitis-related arthritis following anti-tumor necrosis factor-alpha blockade with etanercept. *J Rheumatol.* 2006;33:1186–1188.

24. Lewkowicz D, Gottlieb AB. Pediatric psoriasis and psoriatic arthritis. *Dermatol Ther.* 2004;17:364–375.

Chapter 4
Systemic Lupus Erythematosus (SLE)

4.1 INTRODUCTION

A prototypic autoimmune disease, SLE typically presents in adolescent females, but it can occur as early as the first year of life. Recent advances in the management of lupus, as well as its end-organ manifestations, have improved the outcome tremendously, such that the 10-year-survival rate is now over 90%. Nevertheless, lupus is associated with significant morbidity from the acute disease related events and treatment side effects (Table 4.1).

4.2 ETIOLOGY

The etiology of SLE is complex and relates to interactions between environmental, genetic and endocrine influences. It is more common in certain ethnic groups (Asian, Hispanic, South Asian, African, and African American), and strongly associated with HLA haplotypes. A subgroup is associated with complement deficiencies. Lupus occurs much more commonly after puberty and in females. This suggests an important role for estrogens, which is supported by animal models. Known environmental influences include sun exposure and certain medications (see Section 4.5). The end result of these interactions is the production of multiple autoantibodies that are both organ-specific and directed against a host of nuclear and cytoplasmic antigens. These antibodies form circulating or in situ immune complexes that deposit in vital organs and recruit complement, inflammatory cells and cytokines, which leads to local inflammation and organ damage. The factors leading to autoantibody production are not well understood. One popular hypothesis is that defective apoptosis (programmed cell death) results in exposure of neoantigens on cell surfaces inciting an immune reaction directed against the self.

4.2.1 Prevalence

Lupus is most common in women of child bearing age, which peaks between 19 and 29 years of age. An overall prevalence has

TABLE 4.1. Long-Term Morbidity in Systemic Lupus Erythematosus

Central nervous system
  Cognitive dysfunction
  Stroke

Cardiovascular
  Premature atherosclerosis
  Heart failure

Renal
  Hypertension
  Dialysis
  Transplantation

Skin
  Alopecia

Psychologic
  Depression

Drug-related
  Cyclophosphamide
    Infertility
    Malignancy
  Corticosteroids
    Avascular necrosis
    Osteoporosis
    Obesity following being Cushingoid
    Striae
    Growth failure
    Cataracts

been estimated of 10 to 20 cases per 100,000 people less than 18 years of age. In the experience of clinical staff at The Hospital for Sick Children (Toronto, Ontario, Canada), girls outnumber boys 5:1,[1] but this changes to 10 to 20 women to 1 man in adulthood.

4.3 NATURAL HISTORY AND DISEASE COURSE

4.3.1 Clinical Manifestations

The clinical manifestations reflect the degree of systemic inflammation as well as the organ system(s) affected. Systemic manifestations, both at the time of diagnosis as well as at a time of disease exacerbations, frequently include fever, anorexia, lethargy, weight loss and fatigue. The diagnosis is based on the presence of multisystem involvement with compatible laboratory abnormalities. The presence of 4 of 11 Classification Criteria for SLE,[2] (see Table 4.2) has both a very high sensitivity and specificity for the diagnosis of pediatric SLE.[3]

TABLE 4.2. ACR Classification Criteria[2]

Criterion	Definition
Malar rash	Fixed erythema, flat or raised, over the malar eminences, tending to spare the nasolabial folds
Discoid rash	Erythematous raised patches with adherent keratotic scaling and follicular plugging; atrophic scarring may result in older lesions
Photosensitivity	Skin rash as a result of unusual reaction to sunlight, by patient history or physician observation
Oral ulcers	Oral or nasopharyngeal ulceration, usually painless, observed by physician
Arthritis	Nonerosive arthritis involving 2 or more peripheral joints, characterized by tenderness, swelling, or effusion
Serositis	Pleuritis: Convincing history of pleuritic pain or rubbing heard by a physician or evidence of pleural effusion Or Pericarditis: Documented by ECG or rub or evidence of pericardial effusion
Renal disorder	Persistent proteinuria >0.5 g/day (or >3+ if quantitation not performed) Or Cellular casts: May be red cell, hemoglobin, granular, tubular, or mixed
Neurologic disorder	Seizures in the absence of offending drugs or known metabolic derangements (e.g., uremia: Ketoacidosis or electrolyte imbalance) Or Psychosis in the absence of offending drugs or known metabolic derangements (e.g., uremia: Ketoacidosis or electrolyte imbalance)

TABLE 4.2. *Continued*

Criterion	Definition
Hematologic disorder	Hemolytic anemia with reticulocytosis Or Leukopenia <4,000/mm³ total, on two or more occasions Or Lymphopenia <1,500/mm³ total, on two or more occasions Or Thrombocytopenia <100,000/mm³ total, in the absence of offending drugs
Immunologic disorder	Positive lupus erythematosus cell preparation Or Anti-DNA antibody to native DNA in normal titer Or Presence of anti-Sm nuclear antigen Or False-positive serologic test for syphilis known to be positive for at least 6 months and confirmed by *Treponema pallidum* immobilization or fluorescent treponemal antibody absorption test
Antinuclear antibody	An abnormal titer of antinuclear antibody by immunofluorescence or an equivalent assay at any point in time and in the absence of drugs known to be associated with drug-induced lupus syndromes

4.3.2 Mucocutaneous

Eruptions of the skin and mucus membranes occur in the majority of patients, usually at presentation, and comprise four of the classification criteria. The "butterfly," or malar rash typically occurs on the cheeks, crosses the bridge of the nose but spares the nasal labial folds (Figure 4.1). Findings range from mild erythema to an "angry-looking" vasculitic eruption, which is frequently spotty and not always a typical butterfly rash. Oral ulcers typically involve the hard palate and are usually painless (Figure 4.2).

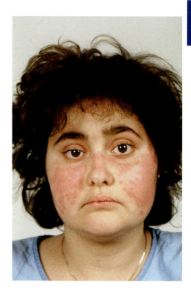

FIGURE 4.1. The "butterfly" or malar rash typically occurs on the cheeks, crosses the bridge of the nose, but spares the nasal labial folds.

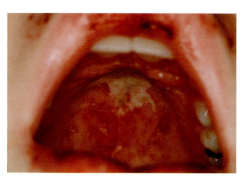

FIGURE 4.2. Oral ulcers, typically involve the hard palate and are usually painless.

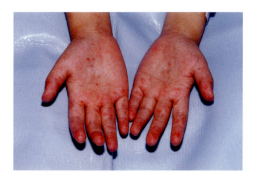

FIGURE 4.3. Additional important mucocutaneous manifestations include peripheral vasculitic changes on the fingers, toes, and earlobes.

Therefore a careful search is warranted. Nasal ulcers may also be asymptomatic, but occasionally lead to septum perforation. Discoid lupus lesions typically occur on the scalp, ears or extensor surfaces. They are hyperkeratotic and purplish with follicular plugging. Discoid lesions are unique in that they may leave permanent scarring and alopecia. Rarely a child will have just discoid lupus without systemic disease. Photosensitivity may result in a blistering rash and sun exposure can precipitate disease flares.

Additional important mucocutaneous manifestations include peripheral vasculitic changes on the fingers, toes and earlobes (Figure 4.3), panniculitis and purpura. Antiphospholipid antibodies are associated with livedo reticularis, a lacy, net-like, reticular rash. Raynaud's phenomenon occurs in 20% of patients and rarely leads to peripheral ischemia or fingertip ulcers.

4.3.3 Musculoskeletal

Arthritis is present in 90% of patients at some time throughout the course. As opposed to the arthritis of juvenile idiopathic arthritis (JIA), the affected joints are usually less swollen but more painful. While erosive disease does not occur, deformities may result from ligamentous stretching. The combination of active disease and treatment with corticosteroids makes osteopenia a major concern and careful attention to bone health must be paid regarding exercise and diet. Pathologic fractures, particularly vertebral, may result in significant morbidity. Corticosteroids may also lead to avascular necrosis, especially involving the femoral heads, humeral heads and tibial plateaus, causing marked pain and loss of motion. Arthralgias and myalgias are common. Myopathy may occur but is rare.

4.3.4 Neurologic

The characteristic neurologic manifestations are seizures and psychosis, but a host of additional signs and symptoms may occur.[4] Perhaps the most common is depression, which usually is reactive to the disease itself, as well as the body altering effect of corticosteroid medications. However, true psychotic depressions may occur. Lupus headache is common and particularly severe. It is unrelieved by standard treatment. It may be related to underlying thrombotic disease. Stroke may result from large vessel inflammation secondary to vasculitis, thrombosis in the antiphospholipid antibody syndrome, or rarely hemorrhage in patients with severe coagulopathy or severe hypertension. Chorea may be the first manifestation of lupus secondary to antiphospholipid antibodies and may be unilateral. Seizures occur in 20% of patients and may result from hypertension, thrombosis, hemorrhage, vasculitis or antibodies against neuronal cells. Transverse myelitis can occur with the antiphospholipid antibody syndrome or it may be due to arteritis and is potentially fatal.

Recently, there has been increased appreciation of an organic brain syndrome associated with lupus and its treatment. This may reflect cerebritis, which results in difficulty concentrating and processing information, or it may be a late effect from lupus and corticosteroid treatment. Magnetic resonance imaging changes of cerebral atrophy are common.

Other neurologic manifestations include peripheral neuropathy and myopathy.

4.3.5 Serositis

Pleuritis, manifesting as pleuritic chest pain with or without pleural effusion, is common and may be unilateral or bilateral. Similarly, pericarditis may lead to central chest pain, worse when leaning forward. The combination of serositis, polyarthritis and fever can be confused with the features of systemic-onset JIA. It is critical to look for features of SLE in patients presenting with isolated serositis.

4.3.6 Renal Disease

Renal disease was the major cause of mortality in patients with lupus, but with earlier diagnosis and newer treatment, the outlook for patients with lupus nephritis has vastly improved.[5] Immune complex deposits in the kidneys result in a variety of pathologic and clinical manifestations. The International Society of Nephrology/Renal Pathology Society *2003 Classification of Lupus Nephritis* is shown in Table 4.3.[6] The histologic abnormalities help determine prognosis and guide treatment.

TABLE 4.3. International Society of Nephrology/Renal Pathology Society 2003 Classification of Lupus Nephritis[6]

Lupus Nephritis Class	
Class I	Minimal mesangial lupus nephritis*
Class II	Mesangial proliferative lupus nephritis[†]
Class III	Focal lupus nephritis[‡]
Class III	(A) Active lesions, focal proliferative lupus nephritis
Class III	(A/C) Active and chronic lesions, focal proliferative and sclerosing lupus nephritis
Class III	(C) Chronic inactive lesions with glomerular scars, focal sclerosing lupus nephritis
Class IV	Diffuse lupus nephritis[§]
Class IV-S	(A) Active lesions, diffuse segmental proliferative lupus nephritis
Class IV-G	(A) Active lesions, diffuse global proliferative lupus nephritis
Class IV-S	(A/C) Active and chronic lesions, diffuse segmental proliferative and sclerosing lupus nephritis
Class IV-G	(A/C) Active and chronic lesions, diffuse global proliferative and sclerosing lupus nephritis
Class IV-S	(C) Chronic inactive lesions with glomerular scars, diffuse segmental sclerosing lupus nephritis
Class IV-G	(C) Chronic inactive lesions with glomerular scars, diffuse global sclerosing lupus nephritis
Class V	Membranous lupus nephritis[¶]
Class V1	Advanced sclerosing lupus nephritis[#]

* Normal glomeruli by light microscopy, but mesangial immune deposits by immunofluorescence.
[†] Purely mesangial hypercellularity of any degree or mesangial matrix expansion by light microscopy, with mesangial immune deposits. A few isolated subepithelial or subendothelial deposits may be visible by immunofluorescence or electron microscopy, but not by light microscopy.
[‡] Active or inactive focal, segmental or global endo—or extracapillary glomeronephritis involving <50% of all glomeruli, typically with focal subendothelial immune deposits, with or without mesangial alterations.
[§] Active or inactive diffuse, segmental or global endo—or extracapillary glomeronephritis involving 50% of all glomeruli, typically with diffuse subendothelial immune deposits, with or without mesangial alterations. This class is divided into diffuse segmental (IV-S) lupus nephritis, when 50% of the involved glomeruli have global lesions. A segmental lesion is defined as a glomerular lesion that involves less than half of the glomerular tuft. This class includes cases with diffuse wire loop deposits, but with little or no glomerular proliferation.
[¶] Global or segmental subepithelial immune deposits or their morphologic sequelae by light microscopy and by immunofluorescence or electron microscopy, with or without mesangial alterations. Class V lupus nephritis may occur in combination with class III or IV in which case both will be diagnosed. Class V lupus nephritis may show advanced sclerosis.
[#] Ninety percent or more of glomeruli globally sclerosed without residual activity.

Importantly, the renal disease may transform from one class to another. Immune complex deposits recruit complement, inflammatory cells and cytokines that result in glomerular damage with necrosis and formation of crescents. Tubulo-interstitial inflammation may develop. Clinical manifestations of renal disease range from none, to mild hematuria, proteinuria and cellular casts to a clinical picture of nephritic syndrome with hypertension, edema and renal failure. Rarely, renal vein thrombosis, usually secondary to the presence of antiphospholipid antibodies or severe nephrotic syndrome, may result in acute hematuria and proteinuria with flank pain. Similarly, renal artery thrombi may cause pain secondary to renal infarction. With current management, less than 10% of patients develop renal failure and require dialysis and transplantation. Renal transplantation, when required, should be performed only once the systemic disease is under control. Recurrent renal disease in a transplanted kidney is rare.

4.3.7 Antiphospholipid Antibody Syndrome (APLS)

Approximately one-third of patients with lupus will develop antiphospholipid antibodies (anticardiolipin, lupus anticoagulant) and some will develop thrombosis. Preliminary classification criteria for APLS have been published.[7] Despite the presence of antibodies that act in the clotting cascade and increase clotting times, patients with APLS form thrombi and both venous and arterial clots may develop. Common presentations include calf deep vein thrombi, stroke, chorea, livedo reticularis, pulmonary emboli and thrombocytopenia.[8] Recurrent miscarriage with fetal loss is another manifestation. Less common manifestations include Budd-Chiari syndrome, renal and splenic infarcts, and Libman-Sachs endocarditis. Rarely, a catastrophic APLS can develop with widespread clotting. This emergency has a high mortality rate. All patients with SLE should be monitored for the presence of these antibodies, and if any clotting occurs, they should probably remain on life long anticoagulation.[9] Less commonly, APLS may occur in isolation, without an associated disease (Primary APLS).

4.3.8 Hematologic

Disorders of hematologic cellular elements, most commonly from antibodies directed either to the blood components themselves or to stem cells, result in hematocytopenias. Autoimmune thrombocytopenic purpura (AITP) may be a presenting feature of SLE and SLE should be suspected, especially in an older patient with AITP who requires more than standard treatment or has extra-hematologic symptoms. Platelet counts may fall to 1–2,000/mm^3. Coombs's positive hemolytic anemia may occur alone or in association with AITP (Evans syndrome) and is a possible manifestation of antiphospholipid antibodies. Both lymphopenia and leukopenia are common. In addition to these lupus-related manifestations, anemia may result from hypersplenism, nutritional deficiency or chronic disease. Thrombocytopenia may be due to APLS. Thrombotic thrombocytopenic purpura in the pediatric population is most commonly related to concurrent SLE or SLE in evolution.

4.3.9 Other Manifestations

4.3.9.1 Cardiac
In addition to pericarditis, myocarditis may rarely develop, with arrhythmias and ventricular dysfunction, and endocarditis, with noninfectious vegetations on the heart valves (a manifestation of APLS).

4.3.9.2 Pulmonary
Rarely, pulmonary disease may predominate and can include pulmonary vasculitis with hemorrhage, interstitial fibrosis, pulmonary hypertension and Shrinking Lung syndrome from diaphragmatic dysfunction.

4.3.9.3 Gastrointestinal
Peritonitis occurs rarely and may be a feature associated with interstitial cystitis. Bowel vasculitis presents with severe abdominal pain and gastrointestinal bleeding. Rarely, pancreatitis is due to lupus and it may also be a side effect of corticosteroids, azathioprine, and mycophenolate mofetil. Hepatic dysfunction with markedly elevated transaminases can be difficult to differentiate from chronic active hepatitis.

4.3.9.4 Sicca Syndrome
Sicca syndrome, with dry mouth and dry eyes, occurs in about 10% of pediatric patients with lupus, especially those who have anti-Ro autoantibodies.

4.3.10 Laboratory Abnormalities
The hallmark of SLE is the presence of autoantibodies, both organ-specific and organ nonspecific, usually with markers of systemic inflammation. Antinuclear antibodies (ANA) are present in virtually all patients with SLE, so much so that the diagnosis is seriously in doubt in their absence. A positive ANA in a patient

suspected of having SLE should promote the search for the specificity of the ANA. Anti-dsDNA antibodies are pathognomonic for SLE and are present in 60% of cases. Their presence correlates with renal disease. Anti-Sm antibodies are also only seen in patients with SLE, but occur in only 25 to 40% of cases. They are frequently seen together with anti-RNP. Antibodies to Ro and La are found in about 30% of patients, and their presence is associated with Sicca syndrome and risk of neonatal lupus in offspring. Rheumatoid Factor, IgM antibodies to IgG, is commonly seen and its presence may lead to a mistaken initial diagnosis of juvenile idiopathic arthritis. Hypocomplementemia, usually indicative of complement consumption (or occasionally complement component deficiency) is reflected by reduced levels of C3, C4 and CH50 and correlates with disease activity. Falling levels, that have been previously normal, suggest an impending disease flare and warrant close observation.

All hematologic cell lines may be reduced together or in isolation. Coombs's positive hemolytic anemia is characteristic and Coombs's test may be positive early on without anemia. Lymphopenia is common and may increase the risk of opportunistic infection. Thrombocytopenia may be present several years before the patient develops more symptoms.

All other tests (urine, blood chemistries, pulmonary function, cardiac tests, imaging) reflect the degree of organ involvement. Characteristically, the erythrocyte sedimentation rate is high and the C-reactive protein (CRP) is normal. The CRP will rise with infections, not lupus flares.

4.3.11 Making the Diagnosis

The key point in making the diagnosis of SLE is to think about it! SLE should be considered in anyone with (1) prolonged marked constitutional symptoms without a diagnosis, (2) multiple organ system disease, (3) polyarthritis in an adolescent, especially a female, (4) unusual presenting features (such as a myocardial infarction in a teenager), and (5) vasculitic rashes. A thorough history and physical examination, a high index of suspicion and appropriate screening laboratory tests will frequently allow the practitioner to make an early diagnosis.

Other autoimmune diseases, malignancy, and chronic infections may be confused with SLE and must always be considered in the differential diagnosis (see Table 4.4).

4.3.12 Treatment

The treatment involves a fine balance between treating the acute events, preventing disease flares, and minimizing treatment-

TABLE 4.4. Differential Diagnosis

Disease Category	Features in Common	Key Differentiators
Other connective tissue diseases	Fever, cytopenia, fatigue, rash	Lack of specific autoantibodies (DNA, Sm), specific features unique to specific diseases (e.g., Gottron's rash of dermatomyositis)
Malignancy	Fever, cytopenia, fatigue, pain, lymphadenopathy, hepatosplenomegaly	Night pain, bone tenderness, normal complement, no urinary changes
Systemic vasculitis	Fever, fatigue, rash	Nodules, calf pain, positive ANCA, bruits
Juvenile idiopathic arthritis	Arthritis, fatigue, fever, rash, lymphadenopathy, marked anemia	Lack of specific autoantibodies (DNA, Sm), normal C3, C4, CH50, no major organ dysfunction
Systemic viral infection	Fever, lymphadenopathy, hepatosplenomegaly, cytopenias	Lack of specific autoantibodies (DNA, Sm), normal C3, C4, CH50

related morbidity. Patients should be seen in a center with experience and expertise in managing childhood SLE. Compliance and lifestyle, especially in adolescents, and the patient and family dynamics are important variables of the treatment plan.

The pharmacologic management should be dictated by the degree of organ system involvement. Virtually all patients require systemic steroids, but the dose is dependent upon the disease activity and should be as low as possible to maintain clinical and laboratory control. At times, the laboratory results do not correlate with the clinical manifestations. In general, laboratory tests should not be treated independently of the clinical findings.

Patients with significant cytopenias or CNS disease will require urgent treatment with high-dose corticosteroids, usually at approximately $60 \, mg/m^2$ (maximum 80 mg) with a slow taper to doses that will keep the disease under control. Many centers use IV methylprednisolone at 30 mg/kg, often repeated on three consecutive days, to gain control of severe disease, and then maintain improvement with 1 to 2 mg/kg oral prednisolone or its equivalent. Corticosteroids are more effective, but also lead to more side effects if given in divided doses. The tapering of corticosteroids must be done carefully and an individualized tapering regimen must be developed. Too rapid a taper may lead to disease flare, transient musculoskeletal pain (pseudorheumatism) or pseudotumor cerebri.

Renal and CNS disease almost always require additional agents. Currently, the ideal choice of agent is unclear. Azathioprine, cyclophosphamide and mycophenolate mofetil all have their proponents, and varying degrees of evidence for and against.[5,10,11] More recently, B cell depletion with a monoclonal antibody (Rituximab) has shown encouraging results, but needs further evaluation. All patients should be treated with hydroxychloroquine to relieve fatigue, reduce disease flares and rash. It may protect against atherosclerosis. Musculoskeletal manifestations and serositis may be managed by nonsteroidal anti-inflammatory drugs or low-dose prednisone. Topical corticosteroids and topical tacrolimus may help skin disease. All patients should avoid excessive sun exposure and use sunblock. If seizures are isolated they may not require any specific therapeutic intervention. Hypertension should be aggressively managed and an ACE inhibitor given to all with any degree of proteinuria, as it seems to decrease the resultant renal damage. Disease related morbidity should be treated in concert with the associated subspecialists.

A general approach to management is listed in Table 4.5.

TABLE 4.5. Systemic Lupus Erythematosus: Treatment

	Minimalist Treatment	May Be Required	Step-Up Treatment, Often Necessary	Occasionally Used	Supportive Treatment
Skin rash	Avoid sun exposure, sun blocks, topical corticosteroids	Low-dose systemic corticosteroids	Thalidomide, vitamin A, cyclosporine, topical tacrolimus		Avoid sun exposure, sun blocks
Arthritis	None, Analgesics, exercise, NSAIDs, Hydroxychloroquine	Low-dose systemic Corticosteroids	Methotrexate		Analgesics, exercise
Renal disease	Low-dose systemic corticosteroids	High-dose systemic corticosteroids, intravenous corticosteroids	Azathioprine, IV "pulse" cyclophosphamide, mycophenolate mofetil	Cyclosporine	Diet, anti-hypertensive
Hematologic disease (cytopenias)	None	Low-dose systemic corticosteroids	Azathioprine, high-dose systemic corticosteroids, intravenous corticosteroids	Vincristine, IV "pulse" cyclophosphamide, IVIG, cyclosporine, dexamethasone, androgens, splenectomy	Transfusions GM-CSF

CNS disease	Rearrange school schedule	Low-dose systemic corticosteroids	High-dose systemic corticosteroids, intravenous corticosteroids	IV "pulse" cyclophosphamide, plasmapheresis	Anti-depressants, anti-psychotics, anti-seizure medications
Bone disease (treatment-related)	Dietary intake of appropriate calcium and vitamin D, exercise	Supplemental calcium and vitamin D	Bisphosphonate		
Anti-phospholipid antibody syndrome	Hydroxychloroquine, avoid oral contraceptives, cardiovascular risk factors, low-dose aspirin	Anti-coagulants		Plasmapheresis	
Fatigue and malaise	Proper rest, exercise	Hydroxychloroquine, low-dose systemic corticosteroids			

Use the lowest amount of the least toxic treatment while maintaining disease under control and preventing long-term complications both from the disease and the treatment!

4.3.13 Prognosis/Outcome

The outcome of patients with SLE has improved dramatically over the last two decades due to a variety of factors, including: earlier diagnosis and institution of treatment; better use of corticosteroids and immunosuppressive medications; better use of supporting medications and sophisticated critical care units. Nevertheless, while the mortality has been reduced substantially such that the 10-year-survival rate is now greater than 90%, morbidity remains substantial. SLE is chronic, and while the disease manifestations can generally be well-controlled, there is always the risk of a disease flare. Flares tend to mimic previous disease manifestations. Factors associated with poor outcome include nonadherence to the treatment regime, significant CNS or cardiac disease, and early hypertension with renal disease.

4.4 NEONATAL LUPUS ERYTHEMATOSUS (NLE)

The term NLE was coined to describe the syndrome in neonates and infants that includes skin rash, heart block, liver disease and cytopenias, and rarely other manifestations, such as bone and CNS disease. The skin and cardiac manifestations are the most frequent. These manifestations result from maternal autoantibodies, most commonly anti-Ro and anti-La, that are transmitted transplacentally and attack fetal and neonatal tissues. For reasons that remain poorly understood, the mother is frequently unaffected, although she produces the autoantibodies. The presence of these autoantibodies puts her at risk, though, for the subsequent development of an autoimmune disease associated with anti-Ro and anti-La antibodies, typically either SLE or Sjögren's Syndrome. Pregnant women with either of these diseases who have anti-Ro and anti-La antibodies are at risk to deliver affected infants, albeit a low risk, less than 5%.[12]

Approximately 50% of affected infants develop an annular erythematous macular skin rash several weeks after birth (Figure 4.4) or after being placed under phototherapy lights. The rash generally disappears by six months of life (concurrent with the disappearance of maternal antibodies from the infant) without complication. Occasionally, at birth there is a raccoon-like periorbital or malar rash that is more deeply erythematous and scaly (Figure 4.5). This may heal with residual scarring, atrophy, hyperpigmentation, and telangiectasiae.

Congenital heart block (CHB) is the second most common manifestation of NLE. It occurs in isolation in about 50% of cases and affects boys more than girls. CHB coexists with cutaneous NLE in about 10% of cases. NLE is the most common cause of

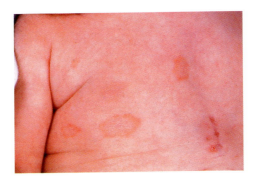

FIGURE 4.4. Scaly annular erythema lesions on the trunk of a baby with NLE: Approximately 50% of affected infants develop an annular erythematous macular skin rash several weeks after birth or after being placed under phototherapy lights.

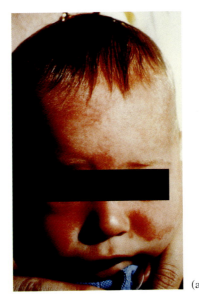

(a)

FIGURE 4.5. (a) Occasionally, at birth there is a raccoon-like periorbital or malar rash that is more deeply erythematous and scaly. (b) ECG changes in NLE, showing AV heart block.

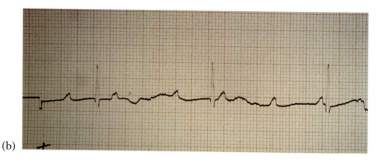

(b)

FIGURE 4.5. *Continued*

"idiopathic" CHB in children, and results for maternal anti-Ro and anti-La antibodies should be obtained in all cases of CHB. The block is at the level of the AV node and is an irreversible third-degree block. While it may be detected in the last part of the second trimester, often it is not recognized until the mother is in labor and the bradycardia is mistaken for fetal distress. Rarely, the bradycardia is so severe that intrauterine congestive heart failure with hydrops fetalis develops. With time, virtually all affected infants will require a pacemaker. Rarely, endocardial fibroelastosis may develop in association with NLE. Intrauterine treatment with maternal dexamethasone may be beneficial.[13]

4.5 DRUG INDUCED LUPUS

Multiple agents have been associated with drug-induced lupus. Clinically this is milder than SLE, usually with less than four criteria, and will remit several months after the inciting agent is stopped. It typically occurs more in elderly Caucasians and has almost an equal frequency between males and females. The most common agent responsible for pediatric drug induced lupus is minocycline, but it is also associated with chlorpromazine, hydralazine, isoniazid, methyldopa, procainamide, and quinidine. Serologically antihistone antibodies are characteristic with the absence of anti-dsDNA and anti-Sm antibodies, and the complement levels are typically normal. Removal of the offending agent should lead to resolution of symptoms, but short-term therapy with NSAIDs, hydroxychloroquine or low-dose corticosteroids may be warranted for symptomatic relief.

References

1. Benseler S, Silverman ED. Systemic lupus erythematosus. *Pediatr Clin North Am.* 2005;52:443–467.

2. Tan EM, Cohen AS, Fries JF et al. The 1982 revised criteria for the classification of systemic lupus erythematosus. *Arthritis Rheum.* 1982;25:1271–1277.
3. Ferraz MB, Goldenberg J, Hilario MO et al. Evaluation of the 1982 ARA lupus criteria data set in pediatric patients. Committees of Pediatric Rheumatology of the Brazilian Society of Pediatrics and the Brazilian Society of Rheumatology. *Clin Exp Rheumatol.* 1994; 12:83–87.
4. Steinlin MI, Blaser SI, Gilday DL et al. Neurologic manifestations of pediatric systemic lupus erythematosus. *Pediatr Neurol.* 1995;13:191–197.
5. Hagelberg S, Lee Y, Bargman J et al. Longterm followup of childhood lupus nephritis. *J Rheumatol.* 2002;29:2635–2642.
6. Weening JJ, D'Agati VD, Schwartz MM et al. The classification of glomerulonephritis in systemic lupus erythematosus revisited. *J Am Soc Nephrol.* 2004;15:241–250.
7. Wilson WA, Gharavi AE, Koike T et al. International consensus statement on preliminary classification criteria for definite antiphospholipid syndrome: report of an international workshop. *Arthritis Rheum.* 1999;42:1309–1311.
8. Ravelli A, Martini A. Antiphospholipid syndrome. *Pediatr Clin North Am.* 2005;52:469–491.
9. Levy DM, Massicotte MP, Harvey E et al. Thromboembolism in pediatric lupus patients. *Lupus.* 2003;12:741–746.
10. Lehman TJ, Onel K. Intermittent intravenous cyclophosphamide arrests progression of the renal chronicity index in childhood systemic lupus erythematosus. *J Pediatr.* 2000;136:243–247.
11. Fine DM. Pharmacological therapy of lupus nephritis. *JAMA.* 2005; 293:3053–3060.
12. Buyon JP, Clancy RM. Neonatal lupus: basic research and clinical perspectives. *Rheum Dis Clin North Am.* 2005;31:299–313.
13. Saleeb S, Copel J, Friedman D, Buyon JP. Comparison of treatment with fluorinated glucocorticoids to the natural history of autoantibody-associated congenital heart block: retrospective review of the research registry for neonatal lupus. *Arthritis Rheum* 1999;42: 2335–2345.

Chapter 5
Juvenile Dermatomyositis

5.1 INTRODUCTION

Juvenile dermatomyositis (JDM) is the most common idiopathic inflammatory myositis in children. Its presentation is unique, with characteristic skin and muscle pathology. JDM is clinically distinct from adult dermatomyositis, because it is a systemic vasculopathy, is not associated with malignancy, overlaps with other childhood inflammatory connective tissue diseases, and generally remits after several years.

5.1.1 Definition

JDM is a vasculopathy of the skin a ld muscle. Typically these patients fulfil the criteria of Bohaen and Peters or that of Rider and Targoff (Table 5.1). However, most rheumatologists do not obtain EMGs or muscle biopsies unless the diagnosis is in doubt. Many will obtain a muscle MRI. If muscle edema is seen on the stir T2 weighted images, inflammation is inferred in the context of the clinical picture.

5.1.2 Epidemiology

Girls are twice to five times as likely to get JDM than boys, most are white, and the peak age of onset is between four and ten years. The incidence in the UK was 1.9 per million souls[1] in young people aged 16 and below, but prevalence is higher in the United States with some clustering of cases (not see in the UK).

5.1.3 Etiology

Multiple theories have been advanced including infectious, maternal microchimerism, genetic (associated with HLA DQA1*0501), and environmental exposures. None have been proven.[2–5]

5.1.4 Clinical Manifestations

There are several different presentations, outlined below:

TABLE 5.1. The Bohan and Peter Diagnostic Criteria and the More Recent Rider and Targoff Criteria to Establish a Diagnosis of JDM

No.	Criteria	Bohan and Peter Criteria	Rider and Targoff Criteria
1	Typical skin rash (heliotrope eyelid rash, Gottron's sign papules over extensor surfaces)	Definite JDM: Criterion 1 plus 3 out of the 4 others (nos. 2–5)	Definite JDM: Criteria 1 plus 3 out of the other 5 (nos. 2–6)
2	Symmetrical proximal muscle weakness	Probable JDM: Criterion 1 plus 2 out of the 4 others (nos. 2–5)	Probable JDM: Criterion 1 plus 2 out of the other 5 (nos. 2–6)
3	Elevation of serum skeletal muscle enzymes (CPK, LDH, ALT, AST, Aldolase)		
4	Specific EMG changes (polyphasic decreased amplitude/duration, positive sharp waves), spontaneous and insertional, high frequency, repetitive discharges	For juvenile polymyositis, criterion 1 is excluded and criteria as from JDM otherwise	This classification adds myositis-specific antibodies as a separate criterion of equal weight
5	Specific muscle biopsy abnormalities (perifascicular degeneration, regeneration, necrosis, phagocytosis, interstitial mononuclear cell infiltrate)		Positive MRI findings may be substituted for criterion 2 or 3
6	Myositis-specific antibodies (anti-synthetase, Mi2, SRP)		

5.1.4.1 Classical JDM

Classical JDM has the characteristic erythematous, often ulcerative, rash over the malar region but it crosses the nasal labial folds and bridge of the nose and spreads onto the forehead, and forms a heliotrope over the outer upper eyelids, Gottron's papules over the knuckles, and a scaly erythematous rash over the elbow and knees. Sometimes keratoderma of the palms and soles is present. Edema of the affected skin and underlying tissues is another feature (Figure 5.1).

There is proximal skeletal muscle weakness especially in the neck, abdominal and hip flexors. Muscle tenderness distinguishes myositis from myopathy due to metabolic, genetic and iatrogenic causes. Joint contractures due to the discomfort and muscle shortening can be the presenting feature. More severe cases will have global weakness, including those of swallowing,

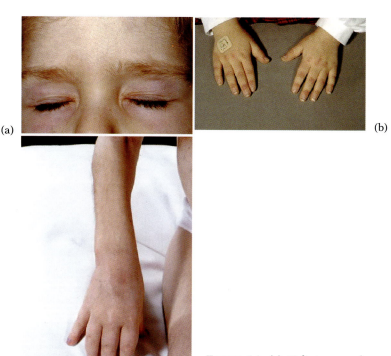

(a)

(b)

(c)

FIGURE 5.1. (a) Heliotrope rash over the eyelids. (b) Gottron's papules over knuckles of the fingers. (c) Soft tissue edema.

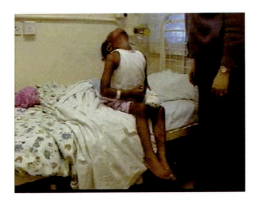

FIGURE 5.2. Proximal muscle weakness, as shown by weak neck flexors.

5

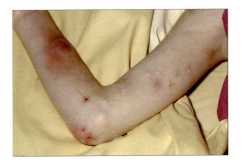

FIGURE 5.3. Calcinosis in JDM.

but the history and detailed muscle testing will reveal the proximal muscle groups as being weakest (Figure 5.2).

Dysphonia often manifests as a higher pitch (bird-like) voice. Involvement of the chest muscles can compromise breathing and artificial ventilation is required in the severest cases. Abdominal pain, difficulty in swallowing and reflux are due to gastrointestinal (GI) dysmotility. More rarely, the myocardium can be affected. Calcinosis is a late manifestation, usually one to two years after onset (Figure 5.3).

5.1.4.2 JDM Sine Myositis

JDM can involve skin alone (thus, sine myositis), although often detailed testing of muscle strength and MRI reveals a proportion of these to have subtle muscle involvement (Figure 5.4).

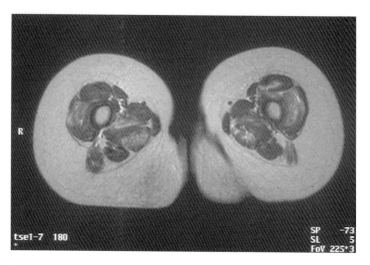

FIGURE 5.4. MRI of the thigh muscle, T2 weighted image, showing patchy inflammation of muscle groups and fasciitis.

5.1.4.3 JDM with Vasculopathy

JDM with vasculopathy is the most severe form. It is associated with classic nailfold capillary changes, showing damaged and blocked small arteries, veins and capillaries. They often have ulcerative skin lesions and multisystem involvement (Figure 5.5). The typical histological appearances are occluded and damaged blood vessels, as well as inflammation. Central nervous system involvement may present with hallucinations or seizures, and MRI of the brain shows characteristic oedematous lesions (Figure 5.6).

Inflammation and blockage of the vasa vasorum of the GI tract can lead to multiple perforations of the whole GI tract (usually the stomach and small intestine). Pulmonary vasculitis leads to spontaneous pneumothorax, and rarely, myocarditis can occur. Therefore, abdominal pain or sudden respiratory distress in the presence of skin ulceration, or other signs of vasculopathy, should be evaluated and treated as an emergency.

This group of patients have a relapsing and chronic course with a high risk of developing calcinosis.

5.1.4.4 JDM with Associated Rheumatic Disease

JDM can present with features of arthritis, SLE, or evolve into systemic sclerosis.

FIGURE 5.5. Skin ulcers in JDM.

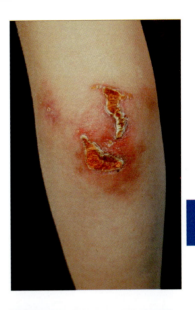

5

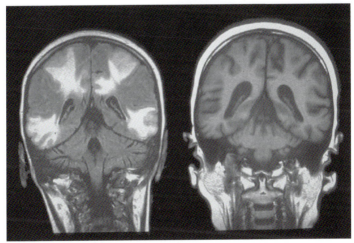

FIGURE 5.6. Brain MRI showing severe edematous areas on the left and complete resolution on the right, after treatment.

5.1.4.5 Polymyositis

Polymyositis is much less common than JDM and many pursue more intensive evaluation given the differential diagnosis (Table 5.2), including muscle biopsy. It can follow a viral infection

TABLE 5.2. Differential Diagnosis for Juvenile Dermatomyositis/ Polymyositis

Conditions	Examples
Conditions that may be associated with rashes:	
Other idiopathic inflammatory Myositis	Focal Myositis, Eosinophilic Myositis, Sarcoid Myositis
Other connective tissue disorders	Systemic Lupus Erythematosus, Mixed Connective Tissue Disease, Scleroderma, other overlap syndromes
Infection-related Myositis	Staphylococcus, Toxoplasmosis, Influenza, Coxsackie
Conditions that are not associated with rashes:	
Neuromuscular disorders	
Muscular dystrophies	
Metabolic and enzyme disorders	Mitochondrial Cytopathies (e.g., McArdle's)
Endocrinopathies	Thyroid and Parathyroid disease, Cu hings
Myasthenia Gravis	
Periodic paralysis	
Myotonia Congenita	

and these tend to remit and not be chronic. Other forms tend to be more chronic and resistant to therapy. Polymyositis tends to be more chronic and resistant to therapy than JDM.

5.1.5 Laboratory Features

The serum levels of muscle enzymes are almost invariably elevated. The creatine kinase (CK) is usually 5 to 20 times normal. Very high levels suggest rhabdomyolysis or muscular dystrophy. The other enzymes, alanine aminotransferase (ALT), lactic dehydrogenase (LDH) and aldolase, should be measured since some patients will have only one or two elevated enzymes. Enzymes are useful for diagnosis in the early stages of the disease, but CK often return to normal as the muscle bulk shrinks due to damage and atrophy. Therefore CK cannot be relied upon to indicate cessation of inflammation. Muscle biopsies are indicated only if the diagnosis is in question, especially if there is no rash or an atypical rash. It is best to have an ultrasound or MRI directed biopsy. EMGs are extremely rarely indicated.

In JDM with vasculopathy, the acute phase markers such as ESR and CRP, are often raised.

In approximately 50% of JDM, there is a positive ANA. If other antinuclear antibodies are present, an overlap with SLE or Scleroderma should be considered, especially in the presence of other clinical features such as Raynaud's or sclerodactyly. Some myositis specific autoantibodies may predict the course; Mi-2 is responsive to treatment, Jo-1 is typical of adult dermatomyositis, and SRP is a poor prognostic indicator.

5.1.6 Diagnosis

Differential diagnoses are listed in Table 5.2. The Bohan and Peter diagnostic criteria and the more recent Rider and Targoff criteria are listed in Table 5.1.

Most clinicians will diagnose JDM if there are at least three of the following features:

- Characteristic skin rashes
- Symmetrical proximal muscle weakness
- Elevation of skeletal muscle enzymes
- MRI evidence of muscle inflammation on T2 echo with fat suppression or ultrasound evidence of muscle inflammation.

5.1.7 Assessment of Disease Activity

Preliminary criteria of assessing disease activity, damage and definition of improvement, have been proposed by the Pediatric Rheumatology International Trials Organization. These are being validated in a prospective study. This tool will allow future therapeutic trials to be assessed and compared.

5.1.8 Treatment

Oral corticosteroid is the standard method of achieving disease control. Long-term corticosteroid orally at 1 to 2 mg/kg is not advisable, because of growth retardation, osteoporosis, and a host of other side effects. Therefore, many pediatric rheumatologists use IV pulse methylprednisolone at 30 mg/kg to achieve induction, followed by lower doses of oral steroids at 0.5 mg/kg/day and the concurrent use of methotrexate or cyclosporine A (Table 5.3). Alternate day steroids do not provide good disease control and the myositis can become more chronic, or progress to a more multisystem vasculopathy. GI disease can impair absorption necessitating all the therapy be given IV

TABLE 5.3. Treatment Algorithm for JDM

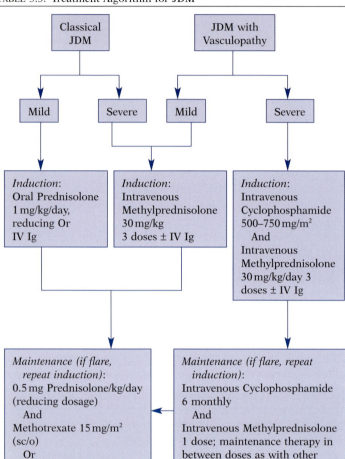

initially. Gastroprotection is necessary, in view of the vasculopathy of the GI tract, and proton pump inhibitors are better for this purpose.

Severe skin disease can be a problem in spite of systemic therapy. Hydroxychloroquine or quinacrine (mepracrine) have been advocated, but the response is not dramatic and trials of topical tacrolimus are in progress. Intravenous immunoglobulins (IVIG) may help.

In the presence of profound myositis or GI or pulmonary vasculopathy, IV cyclophosphamide has been used in addition to IV methylprednisolone.[7] IVIG has a dramatic effect on some patients. Experimental therapies include anti-TNF and autologous stem cell transplants.

Physiotherapy is critical in the management of JDM, as soon as the inflammation is under control, to preserve range of motion and regain strength. Physiotherapist guided exercise to lengthen and strengthen muscles does not increase muscle inflammation.[8] Thus, patients are likely to achieve better function if appropriate physiotherapy is instituted and the patient is not put to bed rest alone. Patients with swallowing difficulty should be nasogatric tube fed until they can safely swallow as documented by cine-esophagram.

5.1.9 Prognosis

Classical JDM usually has a monocyclic course. Relapsing JDM is usually associated with vasculopathy. Relapse of classical JDM can occur many years after remission and after the patient has come off treatment.

If there is severe muscle damage during the disease, function and strength will be compromised. The CK can rise as a result of daily sporting activities, rather than as a result of myositis. In such a situation, MRI of proximal muscle groups can help assess the reason for the raised CK and avoid unnecessary steroid therapy.

Calcinosis of the soft tissue usually indicates severe disease and is associated with significant muscle damage. This can regress once the disease is in remission but may take years. Surgical removal of lumps can be helpful to prevent skin ulcerations at bony prominences. There is no medical treatment to reduce the calcinosis, but it is worth noting that it can be prevented by early diagnosis and aggressive induction of remission.

5.2 KEY POINTS

- Rash and muscle weakness of specific distribution provide the diagnostic clue.
- Be alert for vasculopathy, especially in the GI tract.
- Aggressive anti-inflammatory therapy can lead to remission and prevent calcinosis.

References

1. Symmons DP, Sills JA, Davis SM. The incidence of juvenile dermatomyositis: results from a nation-wide study. *Br J Rheumatol.* 1995;34: 732–736.

2. Artlett CM, Ramos R, Jiminez SA et al. Chimeric cells of maternal origin in juvenile idiopathic inflammatory myopathies. Childhood Myositis Heterogeneity Collaborative Group. *Lancet.* 2000; 356:2155–2156.
3. Reed AM, Picornell YJ, Harwood A et al. Chimerism in children with juvenile dermatomyositis. *Lancet.* 2000;356:2156–2157.
4. Reed AM. Stirling JD. Association of the HLA-DQA1*0501 allele in multiple racial groups with juvenile dermatomyositis. *Hum Immunol.* 1995;44:131–135.
5. Pachman LM, Liotta–Davis MR, Hong DK et al. TNF-alpha-308A allele in juvenile dermatomyositis: association with increased production of tumor necrosis factor ALPHA, disease duration, and pathologic calcifications. *Arthritis Rheum.* 2000;43:2368–2377.
6. Ruperto N, Ravelli A, Murray KJ et al. Preliminary core sets of measures for disease activity and damage assessment in juvenile systemic lupus erythematosus and juvenile dermatomyositis. *Rheumatology (Oxford).* 2003;42:1452–1459.
7. Riley P, Maillard SM, Wedderburn LR et al. Intravenous cyclophosphamide pulse therapy in juvenile dermatomyositis: a review of efficacy and safety. *Rheumatology (Oxford).* 2004;43:491–496.
8. Maillard SM, Jones R, Owens C et al. Quantitative assessment of MRI T2 relaxation time of thigh muscles in juvenile dermatomyositis. *Rheumatology (Oxford).* 2004;43:603–608.

Chapter 6
Scleroderma

6.1 INTRODUCTION

The scleroderma group of diseases are all characterized by the presence of hard skin. One classification of the various forms of scleroderma is listed in Table 6.1. Successful treatment of these disorders has lagged behind that of many of the other rheumatic diseases.

6.2 ETIOLOGY AND PATHOGENESIS

Observations on the pathogenesis of scleroderma include (a) excessive production of collagen and extracellular matrix by fibroblasts, not only in the skin but also in vital organs and around blood vessels; this is often preceded by an initial inflammatory phase (especially in localized scleroderma, as seen clinically from biopsy and thermography); (b) endothelial cell injury with upregulation of vascular adhesion molecules, and (c) abnormalities of immune regulation, such as altered cytokine and chemokine balance, T-cell activation, and the presence of autoantibodies.[1] Also, interactions between environmental exposures and the individual genetic makeup are likely to be important contributors to the pathogenesis of these diseases. Maternal microchimerism may also play a role in disease pathogenesis, but this remains unclear at the present time.[2]

6.3 EPIDEMIOLOGY

6.3.1 Systemic Sclerosis (SSc)

SSc usually constitutes less than 1% of most pediatric rheumatology clinic populations. In adults, the highest reported incidence is 1.9 per 100,000 with a prevalence of approximately 24 per 100,000.[3] Females are affected much more commonly than males.

TABLE 6.1. Scleroderma and Scleroderma-Like Disorders

Systemic sclerosis
  Diffuse
  Limited
  Overlap syndromes

Localized scleroderma
  Morphea
  Linear Scleroderma
  En coup de Sabre
  Parry–Romberg syndrome

Scleroderma-like disorders
  Graft versus host disease
  Drug/toxin induced
  Diabetic Cheiroarthropathy
  Phenylketonuria
  Premature aging syndromes

TABLE 6.2. Raynaud's Phenomenon

Primary

Secondary
  Connective Tissue Disease
    Scleroderma
    Mixed Connective Tissue Disease
    Systemic Lupus Erythematosus
    Dermatomyositis
    Overlap syndromes
  Mechanical Obstruction
    Thoracic Outlet Syndrome
    Cervical Rib
  Drug/toxin induced
  Cryoglobulinemia
  Polycythemia

Vibratory worker

6.4 CLINICAL FEATURES

The diagnosis is usually suspected in a child who presents with Raynaud's phenomenon (characteristic triphasic color change of distal body parts on exposure to cold or stress: white to blue to red) and other systemic manifestations. The differential diagnosis of Raynaud's phenomenon is large (Table 6.2). The absence of Raynaud's phenomenon should always lead one to question

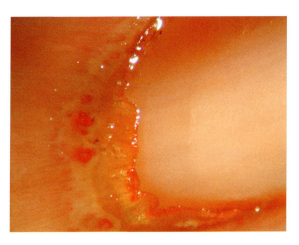

FIGURE 6.1. Abnormal nailfold capillary microscopy.

6

the diagnosis of SSc. Children presenting with isolated Raynaud's phenomenon alone may go on to develop scleroderma. Hints that the Raynaud's phenomenon is likely to evolve to another illness include abnormal nail fold vasculature (Figure 6.1) and the presence of a positive antinuclear antibody (ANA).[4]

The earliest skin manifestation of SSc is nonpitting inflammatory edema of the hands, which results in restrictive range of motion of the hands. With time, this evolves to skin thickening and tightness with an inability to lift the skin. Clinical methods to quantify skin thickening have been validated in adults but not in children.[5] Progressive thickening and tightness of the skin result in joint contractures and an inability to fully open the mouth (Figure 6.2). In addition, there is a progressive loss of hair follicles. Other skin manifestations include abnormal nail folds and calcinosis over the bridge of the nose (Figure 6.3), telangiectasia, and areas of skin breakdown over pressure points. Areas of hyperpigmentation and hypopigmentation can result in a "salt and pepper" appearance. The distribution of thickening differs in the two major types of SSc (diffuse and limited). Involvement proximal to the wrist and ankles, and involvement of the trunk, is more characteristic of diffuse disease which has a higher rate of internal organ involvement and earlier clinical manifestations of internal organ dysfunction. Limited SSc (formerly known as CREST Syndrome) progresses much more slowly, but there is a greater risk of the late development of pulmonary hypertension.

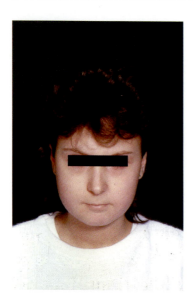

FIGURE 6.2. Tight skin on the face of a 14-year-old girl with diffuse systemic sclerosis.

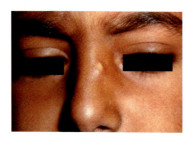

FIGURE 6.3. Calcinosis over the nasal bridge in an 8-year-old boy with systemic sclerosis.

Musculoskeletal involvement is common. Fibrosis of the joint capsule and thickening of the synovium results in joint contractures, a problem exacerbated by the thickened and tight skin around the joint. The joints may be tender but are not usually swollen. A subclinical myopathy, with minimal weakness and mild elevation of serum levels of muscle enzymes is common. More significant muscle involvement can occasionally occur, especially when there is an overlap with the myositis syndromes. Another characteristic feature, tendon friction rubs, can be felt and heard over the wrists and ankles.

Gastrointestinal involvement is a major cause of morbidity (Table 6.3). Dysphagia results from poor esophageal peristalsis

TABLE 6.3. Gastrointestinal Manifestations

Dysphagia
Esophageal reflux
Bacterial overgrowth with malabsorption
Megacolon with constipation

TABLE 6.4. Pleuropulmonary Manifestations

Pleural effusion
Inflammatory alveolitis
Interstitial fibrosis
Pulmonary hypertension

secondary to esophageal fibrosis. Dysfunction of the lower esophageal sphincter results in acid reflux and the potential for the development of reflux esophagitis. Dysmotility of the small intestine may lead to stasis, bacterial overgrowth and malabsorption with diarrhea. Finally, severe constipation and megacolon occasionally occur.

Renal disease, formerly the major cause of mortality, is now more manageable with the advent of angiotensin converting enzyme inhibitors. Renal vasculopathy may lead to the development of "scleroderma kidney," which usually presents with hypertension. The hypertension may be preceded by proteinuria. Glomerular disease is unusual.

The major current cause of mortality results from pulmonary involvement, which can take several forms (Table 6.4). The more common is interstitial lung disease. This begins as an inflammatory alveolitis, which evolves to interstitial fibrosis. It is critical to discover the lung disease in its early stage when it may still be responsive to treatment. The second most common form of pulmonary disease is pulmonary hypertension, which can occur in isolation as part of the vasculopathy of scleroderma, or secondary to the interstitial lung disease. Symptoms include dyspnea and hypoxemia. This can usually be detected by echocardiography. Finally, pleuritis with or without pleural effusion may also occur. Early symptoms of pulmonary involvement include dry cough, followed by progressive dyspnea on exertion. On examination, dry rales are common and may be associated with reduced chest expansion.

The heart is also commonly affected. Pericarditis with small pericardial effusions is very common. Involvement of the cardiac microvasculature leads to tiny areas of microinfarcton, which can eventually result in a cardiomyopathy. Involvement of the conducting system by fibrosis can result in bundle branch block or other arrhythmias.

Other systemic involvement includes periodontal ligaments with dental loosening, bony resorption, rare neuropathies (e.g., trigeminal), Sjögren's syndrome and thyroid involvement.

6.5 INVESTIGATIONS

Laboratory features can be divided into those that are nonspecific and reflect the presence and degree of organ involvement, and those that are more specific to the different forms of scleroderma (Table 6.5). Laboratory signs of systemic inflammation are generally absent, except early on in the disease where the erythrocyte sedimentation rate (ESR) and other markers of acute inflammation may be elevated. Anemia may result from poor diet, malabsorption or chronic disease. Signs of endothelial activation are reflected in a raised von Willebrand factor antigen. Mild elevations of serum levels of muscle enzymes accompany the scleroderma myopathy and these are significantly raised in overlap syndromes. It is important to do screening and monitoring of the pulmonary function tests. Early disease is reflected in a reduced DLCO, while progressive fibrosis is shown by a reduced residual volume and forced vital capacity and FEV1. High resolution, thin-section CT scan of the lungs, is critically important in the evaluation of patients.[6] Early alveolitis is shown by the presence of ground-glass appearance, primarily in the lung bases, before the development of fibrosis. The presence of pulmonary hypertension may be sought by cardiac echocardiography, although at intermediate levels of pulmonary hypertension a cardiac catheterization may be required. Renal abnormalities

TABLE 6.5. Suggested Laboratory Investigations

System/Organ	Investigation
Immune	ANA, RF, anti-Scl 70, anti-centromere
Renal	U/A for proteinuria
Cardiac	EKG (rhythm), Echocardiogram (pulmonary hypertension)
Pulmonary	PFTs with DLCO, chest X-ray, high-resolution CT scan
GI	Upper GI series (reflux)

are uncommon until proteinuria indicates the onset of sclero-derma kidney.

Serologic abnormalities are common and help classify patients. Nonspecific antinuclear antibodies, usually with a speckled or nucleolar pattern, are seen in 75% of patients, and rheumatoid factor positivity in a minority of patients. The speci-ficity of the ANA is important. The presence of anti SCL-70 (antitopoisomerase I) correlates with the diffuse SSc, and anti-centromere antibodies with limited SSc. Other autoantibodies may occur.

6.6 COURSE AND OUTCOME

The course of SSc is usually characterized by skin tightening with eventual softening over time. Unfortunately, organ dys-function is progressive over several years, at which point there is either stabilization or death. The outcome is determined by the rate of progression of internal organ manifestations in the first few years after presentation. In the largest reported survey of patients with SSc, 8 of 135 patients died (5 from heart failure, 1 from renal failure, 1 from sepsis and 1 from unknown causes), but in general, the outcome was better than in adult SSc.[7] Severe early skin thickening is a poor prognostic indicator in adults with SSc.

6.7 TREATMENT

Treating patients with scleroderma has been very frustrating for all practitioners, although some recent progress has been made. Most important have been the advances in treating end-organ manifestations. Treatment should be considered in terms of (1) the disease process itself, (2) end organ manifestations, and (3) general supportive measures.

Disease Process. To date, no treatment has been proven defini-tively to alter the course of SSc.[8] Immunomodulatory agents, which may be effective include methotrexate, mycophenolate mofetil, cyclophosphamide, and antithymocyte globulin. Further studies are required and are ongoing. At least one pediatric patient has had resolution of disease following autologous stem cell transplantation,[9] but this is still considered experimental.

End-Organ Manifestations and Supportive Treatment. The mor-bidity of SSc has been dramatically altered due to the availabil-ity of agents to treat the disease manifestations. Table 6.6 lists the treatment options for the various end-organ manifestations.

TABLE 6.6. Treatment of End-Organ Manifestations

Manifestation	Supportive Measure	Pharmacologic Treatment
Raynaud's phenomenon	Keep warm	Peripheral vasodilators (e.g., nifedipine, losartan)
Reflux esophagitis	Small meals, elevate head of bed, do not lie supine after eating	Proton pump inhibitors
Renal disease	Appropriate diet	ACE inhibitor
Pulmonary interstitial fibrosis		Trial of glucocorticoids and cyclophosphamide
Pulmonary hypertension		Trial of endothelin receptor antagonist (bosentan)

TABLE 6.7. Preliminary Criteria for the Classification of Systemic Sclerosis[10]

Major criterion
    Proximal scleroderma: Typical sclerodermatous skin changes
        involving areas proximal to the metacarpophalangeal or
        metatarsophalangeal joints

Minor criteria
    Sclerodactyly
    Digital pitting scars
    Bibasilar pulmonary fibrosis

Definite scleroderma requires the presence of the major criterion or 2 minor criteria.

6.7.1 Making the Diagnosis

Preliminary criteria for the classification of systemic sclerosis have been established (Table 6.7), but these were developed for adults.[10] Recently, classification criteria for childhood systemic sclerosis have been proposed, (Table 6.8) and are currently under study.[11]

There are several clinical scenarios in which systemic sclerosis should be suspected even prior to the development of skin changes, as listed in Table 6.9.

TABLE 6.8. Preliminary Classification Criteria for Systemic Sclerosis in Children[11]

Major criteria
  Raynaud's phenomenon
  Sclerosis/induration
  Scelrodactyly

Minor criteria
  Vascular
  Musculoskeletal
  Gastrointestinal
  Respiratory
  Cardiac
  Renal
  Neurologic
  Serology

Presence of sclerosis/induration and at least 2 minor criteria.
Presence of Raynaud's phenomenon and sclerosis/induration and at least 1 minor criterion.
Presence of Raynaud's phenomenon and sclerosis/induration and at least 2 minor criteria.

TABLE 6.9. When to Consider Scleroderma

Raynaud's phenomenon in the presence of a positive ANA and/or abnormal nailfold capillaries
Polyarthritis with minimal effusions
Unexplained pulmonary fibrosis
Severe gastroesophageal reflux
Unexplained myopathy

6.7.2 Localized Scleroderma

In children, localized forms of scleroderma are much more common than systemic ones and, while generally much milder, they can be associated with localized abnormalities that can have serious consequences.[12] Like systemic disease, the unifying feature is hardening of the skin. Yet some forms considered to be part of LS are associated with atrophy rather than hardening, and often the initial firm phase gives way to softening with atrophy. Although the classifications include many forms, only the most common ones will be described here.

6.7.3 Plaque Morphea

The most characteristic lesion of morphea is a plaque involving the trunk (Figure 6.4). This usually begins as a firm-ivory colored

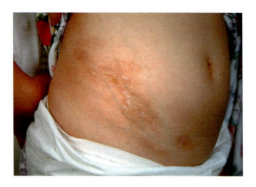

FIGURE 6.4. Plaque morphea lesion involving the trunk.

oval lesion which may be up to several centimeters in size. Symptoms may include tingling or itching. The center is usually surrounded by a reddish-lilac color ring that suggests the process is active and inflammatory. The lesion often expands over several years, but eventually softens spontaneously. As part of the healing process, atrophy with hyperpigmentation commonly evolve. When there are more than three lesions, the disorder is known as Generalized Morphea. A variant, Disabling Pansclerotic Morphea, is characterized by diffuse thickening, which involves all extremities and the trunk. This may result in severe contractures and restriction in chest wall movement.

6.7.4 Linear Scleroderma
Over 50% of children with localized forms of scleroderma will have bands of firm sclerotic tissue in a linear distribution, classified as Linear Scleroderma (Figure 6.5). The location will determine the impact and course. If the lesion crosses joints, it may result in contractures and loss of motion. It also may affect the growth, both circumferential as well as linear of the extremity and occasionally result in a withered, nonfunctional limb. Muscle atrophy and shortening of the extremity are not uncommon.

When linear scleroderma affects the face, the disorder is known as either scleroderma "en coup de sabre", or progressive hemifacial atrophy, also known as Parry–Romberg Syndrome. En coup de sabre lesions occur on the forehead, usually in paramedian distribution, and often extend upward into the scalp with associated localized alopecia (Figure 6.6). Early on, the band is firm and "cuts into" the forehead and scalp with localized

FIGURE 6.5. Linear scleroderma lesion.

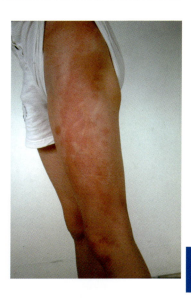

6

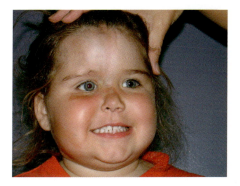

FIGURE 6.6. En coup de sabre scleroderma lesion.

atrophy. It may extend through muscle and bone and result in defects in the skull vault. The band may cross the eye and "tent" the nasal ala. Uveits and orbital inflammatory masses can occur. Deeper involvement may irritate the cerebral cortex and result in seizures. Cerebral calcifications are common, but their significance is uncertain. The lesion may extend lower to involve the lips, tongue, maxillary and mandibular bones. Patients with Parry–Romberg Syndrome have significant facial deformities, which progress over time as the unaffected side continues its

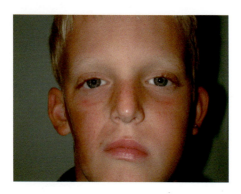

FIGURE 6.7. Parry–Romberg Syndrome.

normal growth (Figure 6.7). Dental abnormalities commonly are associated.

6.8 DIAGNOSIS

The diagnosis is made clinically by recognizing the characteristic lesions. When there is doubt, a skin biopsy showing thickening of the collagen bundles will confirm the diagnosis. Laboratory abnormalities can include mild elevation of the ESR, hypergammaglobulinemia, eosinophilia and a positive ANA and rheumatoid factor. However, all may be normal even in active disease.

6.9 TREATMENT

As with systemic disease, no systemic treatments have been proven effective in patients with LS. Since the natural history is for these lesions to soften with time, the risk of treatment must be carefully weighed against benefit. For plaque morphea, treatment with topical corticosteroids or calcipotriene[13] may be effective. Deep tissue massage may also be helpful. When lesions are appearing rapidly, crossing joint lines, or have the potential to result in serious cosmetic deformity and functional disability, systemic treatments are often considered early to suppress the inflammatory phase, with a view to halt the progression to growth abnormalities and fibrosis. Currently, a combination of short-term corticosteroid and longer-term methotrexate (approximately 15 mg/m² per week) is frequently used.[14]

References

1. Artlett CM. Immunology of systemic sclerosis. *Front Biosci.* 2005;10:1707–1719.
2. Jimenez SA, Artlett CM. Microchimerism and systemic sclerosis. *Curr Opin Rheumatol.* 2005;17:86–90.
3. Mayes MD, Lacey JV Jr, Beebe-Dimmer J et al. Prevalence, incidence, survival, and disease characteristics of systemic sclerosis in a large US population. *Arthritis Rheum.* 2003;48:2246–2255.
4. Duffy CM, Laxer RM, Lee P et al. Raynaud's syndrome in childhood. *J Pediatr.* 1989;114:73–78.
5. Furst DE, Clements PJ, Steen VD et al. The modified Rodnan skin score is an accurate reflection of skin biopsy thickness in systemic sclerosis. *J Rheumatol.* 1998;25:84–88.
6. Seely JM, Jones LT, Wallace C et al. Systemic sclerosis: using high-resolution CT to detect lung disease in children. *AJR Am J Roentgenol.* 1998;170:691–697.
7. Foeldvari I, Zhavania M, Birdi N et al. Favourable outcome in 135 children with juvenile systemic sclerosis: results of a multi-national survey. *Rheumatology (Oxford).* 2000;39:556–559.
8. Zulian F. Scleroderma in children. *Pediatr Clin North Am.* 2005;52: 521–545.
9. Martini A, Maccario R, Ravelli A et al. Marked and sustained improvement two years after autologous stem cell transplantation in a girl with systemic sclerosis. *Arthritis Rheum.* 1999;42:807–811.
10. Preliminary criteria for the classification of systemic sclerosis (scleroderma). Subcommittee for scleroderma criteria of the American Rheumatism Association Diagnostic and Therapeutic Criteria Committee. *Arthritis Rheum.* 1980;23:581–590.
11. Zulian F et al. *Arthritis Rheum.* In Press.
12. Murray KJ, Laxer RM. Scleroderma in children and adolescents. *Rheum Dis Clin North Am.* 2002;28:603–624.
13. Cunningham BB, Landells ID, Langman C et al. Topical calcipotriene for morphea/linear scleroderma. *J Am Acad Dermatol.* 1998; 39:211–215.
14. Uziel Y, Feldman BM, Krafchik BR et al. Methotrexate and corticosteroid therapy for pediatric localized scleroderma. *J Pediatr.* 2000;136:91–95.

Chapter 7
Overlap Syndromes

7.1 INTRODUCTION

Many patients present with clinical and laboratory signs and symptoms that are compatible with several of the classic Connective Tissue Disease (CTD), such as juvenile idiopathic arthritis (JIA), Systemic Lupus Erythematosus (SLE), Juvenile Dermatomyositis (JDM), and Systemic Sclerosis (SSc). These children, who have overlapping features of several CTDs, are said to have "overlap syndromes" or "undifferentiated connective tissue diseases." Patients may remain with overlapping features for many years, or their clinical picture may evolve into one of the more classic CTDs. Two overlap CTDs are better defined in terms of having diagnostic criteria and characteristic serologic features: mixed connective tissue disease (MCTD) and Sjögren's syndrome (SS).

7.2 MIXED CONNECTIVE TISSUE DISEASE

MCTD is a disease whose manifestations include features of SLE, JIA, JDM, and SSc, with a high titer antinuclear antibody and speckled pattern on immunofluorescence, together with specific autoantibodies directed against the U1RNP component of the extractable nuclear antigen (ENA) complex (Table 7.1). MCTD, like other autoimmune diseases, has certain immunogenetic associations, suggesting that these patients are "genetically pre-determined" to develop the disease. An inciting environmental agent(s) is likely critical to trigger the development of autoantibodies and disease manifestations. A variety of diagnostic criteria have been proposed for MCTD, but none have been validated in children.[1]

Most commonly, early symptoms include swelling with edema of the hands (Figure 7.1) and Raynaud's phenomenon. The remaining clinical manifestations are determined by which component of the "overlapping" disease is playing the most prominent role. For instance, it may be the rash and proximal

TABLE 7.1. Mixed Connective Tissue Disease*

A disease characterized by features of several autoimmune
   connective tissue diseases, SLE, JIA, JDM, and scleroderma
High-titer antinuclear antibodies with a speckled pattern on
   immunofluorescence antibodies to U1RNP

*The presence of other specific antinuclear antibodies in high titer
should exclude the diagnosis of MCTD.

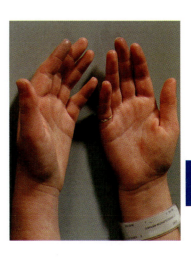

FIGURE 7.1. Picture showing
"sausage fingers" seen in early
MCTD.

muscle weakness of JDM; esophageal disturbance and lung
disease of scleroderma; the malar rash and serositis of SLE; or
the polyarthritis of JIA. Severe glomerulonephritis and thrombocytopenia are uncommon unless the MCTD evolves towards
"full-blown" SLE, in which case additional autoantibodies
usually develop.

7.2.1 Prevalence
MCTD is uncommon in children and represents less than 1% of
most pediatric rheumatology clinic populations. It occurs most
commonly in adolescence with a female to male ratio of approximately 5:1.[1] The usual age of onset is in the early adolescent
years, but can occur in children as young as five years of age.

7.3 NATURAL HISTORY AND DISEASE COURSE
Features at onset often include puffiness of the fingers and hands
(Figure 7.1). Skin signs of SLE and JDM and proximal muscle
weakness are seen early in the course. The myositis may not be

as severe as in JDM. Arthritis is an early feature, frequently persists and can lead to deformities with or without erosions. Arthritis may involve large and small joints, typically in a symmetrical pattern. Tight skin may contribute to joint contractures.

Raynaud's phenomenon, another of the characteristic early features present in the majority of cases of MCTD, usually persists throughout the course, and is often severe with potential to leave digital scarring.

Pulmonary function abnormalities are common throughout the course, although usually asymptomatic at onset. However, with time interstitial lung disease may develop and, more rarely, pulmonary hypertension occurs. Patients must be monitored closely for the development of either of these two potentially fatal disorders (see Chapter 6).

Renal disease is not common, unless the patient pursues a course more akin to SLE, in which case manifestations of glomerulonephritis and nephrotic syndrome can occur. Rarely, renal failure develops.

Other clinical manifestations include those that may occur in the diseases that contribute to the overlap. Pleuritis and pericarditis, both representing contributions of SLE or scleroderma, can occasionally occur. The classic cutaneous features of JDM, such as Gottron's popula and heliotrope rash (Figure 7.2) may be seen. The gastrointestinal manifestations associated with scleroderma, such as dysphagia and reflux, often develop with time. Sicca symptoms are common. Central nervous manifestations are uncommon, unless the MCTD is dominated by features of SLE. Leukopenia and thrombocytopenia are frequent findings.

7.3.1 Diagnosis

The diagnosis is based on the combination of features of various classic autoimmune connective tissue diseases, together with the laboratory features of high titer ANA in speckled pattern and the presence of antibodies to U1RNP. No other ANA specificity should be present. It should be noted that antibodies to U1RNP may also occur, in lower titer, in patients with SLE and scleroderma.

7.3.2 Course and Outcome

Patients must be followed closely for evolution of organ system dysfunction and failure, especially the lungs and kidneys. A small number of patients may go into a full remission and not require medication.[2] However, mortality is reported in the range of 3 to 28%. Deaths have resulted from infection, and are likely related

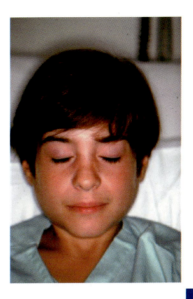

FIGURE 7.2. A 14-year-old girl with overlap syndrome who complained of joint pain as well as sudden onset of pain and swelling over the angle of both jaws: Note the heliotropic discoloration over the eyelids and bilateral parotid swelling typical of Sjögren's Syndrome.

7

to immunosuppression needed to manage the disease. Death has also been reported due to severe renal disease, pulmonary hypertension and myocarditis. The course is dictated by whether the disease evolves into a lupus-like or scleroderma-like process.

Overall, approximately 75% of patients have a favourable outcome. There are important HLA associations which may be associated with course and outcome.

7.3.3 Treatment
There is nothing specific to the treatment of MCTD other than careful attention to vital organ involvement and provision of ongoing family-centered care and psychosocial support. The reader should refer to the specific chapters for treatment of the various clinical manifestations of MCTD.

7.4 SJÖGREN'S SYNDROME
Sjögren's syndrome is an overlap syndrome, which may occur as part of an underlying autoimmune CTD (in which case it is known as secondary SS) or in isolation, also known as primary SS[3] (Table 7.2). Secondary SS is more common, and is seen in children most commonly with JIA, SLE, scleroderma, and MCTD. SS is characterized clinically by the "Sicca complex" of dry eyes and dry mouth, in association with anti-Ro and anti-La antibodies (also known as anti-SSA and anti-SSB, respectively).

TABLE 7.2. Sjögren's Syndrome

Keratoconjcunctivitis sicca (dry eyes and dry mouth)
Plus
Autoantibodies (anti-Ro, anti-La)

Sjögren's Syndrome is considered *primary* if not associated with any other connective tissue disease and *secondary* when it occurs together with another CTD (most commonly, SLE; also, MCTD, scleroderma, and JIA).

The pathology of SS is characterized by lymphocytic inflammation of exocrine glands, especially the salivary and lacrimal glands. The inciting agent that results in this attack is unknown; several authors have postulated an underyling viral etiology. Other affected glandular tissues may include the renal tubules and bile canaliculi with resultant clinical manifestions of renal tubular acidosis and primary biliary cirrhosis. The role of the autoantibodies in pathogenesis is unknown but their presence is almost universal. Patients with SS generally have the immunogentic phenotype HLADR3, DQw1, and DQw2.

7.4.1 Prevalence

SS is rare in childhood. Fewer that 150 cases have been reported. Secondary SS is more common and is associated with CTDs whose incidence is increased in adolescence, SS is seen more commonly in late adolescence, but it has been reported in children as young as five years of age. The criteria proposed for adult SS may not be relevant for children, but diagnostic criteria have recently been proposed for juvenile Sjögren's syndrome.[4]

7.5 NATURAL HISTORY AND DISEASE COURSE

The clinical manifestations relate to the sicca complex primarily and to glandular inflammation. The most common presenting feature in children is recurrent parotitis that is not responsive to antibiotics (Figure 7.2). With time, recurrent lymphocytic infiltration of the salivary glands will result in destruction of ductal tissue and reduced salivary flow, which will result in persistent dry mouth. On examination, there is a poor saliva pool under the tongue and the tongue blade often sticks to the tongue. Patients have difficulty initating swallowing ("upper" dysphagia) and often have to have water by their bedside at night. Dental caries become a significant problem. Ocular dryness results in photophobia with a feeling of "sand" in the eye. In adult women, vaginal dryness with dyspareunia is a major problem. If the SS is secondary to another CTD, symptoms and signs of that CTD may dominate. However, extraglandular signs and symptoms occur in a significant percentage of children with primary SS, including hematologic (primarily neutropenia), cutaneous vasculitis, arthritis/arthralgias, peripheral lymphadenopathy, peripheral neuropathy and CNS involvement. A persistent metabolic acidosis, secondary to renal tubular acidosis may occur and can affect growth. B-cell lymphoma, which does occur in adults with SS, has not been reported as an association in pediatric SS.

7.5.1 Diagnosis

SS is frequently accompanied by significant hypergammaglobulinemia, positive rheumatoid factor in high titer, positive ANA in high titer, and anti-Ro and anti-La antibodies. Elevated levels of serum amylase are common. Importantly, antibodies to dsDNA, and cardiolipin are negative, as is ANCA, and serum complement levels are normal. Ocular dryness can be confirmed by a positive Schirmer's Test (placing a strip of filter paper in the ocular sac and observing the degree of wetting over five minutes); <5 mm is considered a positive test. A Rose Bengal corneal stain may demonstrate corneal erosions resulting from ocular dryness. Xerostomia can be investigated by salivary scan, showing reduced salivary flow. A biopsy of minor salivary glands, demonstrating lymphocytic infiltration, may occasionally be necessary, especially when excluding other causes of parotitis. Malignancy and sarcoidosis should always be considered in the differential diagnosis.

7.5.2 Course and Outcome

Fortunately, the outcome of children with primary SS is good, although symptomatic treatment is necessary to improve their quality of life. For extra glandular manifestations with life-threatening potential, treatment with corticosteroids, or more rarely, cyclophosphamide (especially for CNS disease) is necessary.

7.5.3 Treatment

Ocular and oral dryness are very troublesome to patients and attention to local hygiene is extremely important. Artificial tears should be used to maintain corneal hydration, and saliva substitutes have also recently become available. Careful attention must be paid to the prevention of dental caries. Oral pilocarpine may help both the oral and ocular sicca symptoms. The treatment of the systemic manifestations is based on the specific organ involvement, and usually includes NSAIDs, hyroxychloroguine, and corticosteroids.

References
1. Mier RJ, Shishov M, Higgins GC et al. Pediatric-onset mixed connective tissue disease. *Rheum Dis Clin North Am.* 2005;31:483–496.
2. Michels H. Course of mixed connective tissue disease in children. *Ann Med.* 1997;29:359–364.
3. Cimaz R, Casadei A, Rose C et al. Primary Sjögren's syndrome in the paediatric age: a multicentre survey. *Eur J Pediatr.* 2003;162:661–665.
4. Bartunkova J, Sediva A, Vencovsky J et al. Primary Sjogren's syndrome in children and adolescents: proposal for diagnostic criteria. *Clin Exp Rheumatol.* 1999;17:381–386.

Chapter 8
Vasculitis

8.1 INTRODUCTION

Vasculitis is an inflammatory and often destructive process of the blood vessels. These diseases are difficult to diagnose as presenting symptoms can be nonspecific and multiple organs are involved. Primary vasculitis denotes inflammation of the blood vessels not associated with other inflammatory disease processes. Many childhood multisystem inflammatory diseases may include components of vasculitis and these are designated as secondary vasculitis. This chapter will concentrate on primary vasculitis. The initial symptoms can be lethargy, skin rash and other constitutional symptoms, or an acute medical emergency with multisystem dysfunction and irritability. A recent international consensus conference of experts agreed to a classification of childhood vasculitis, because childhood onset vasculitis has many unique features compared to adult forms (Table 8.1).[1] This is a modification of the Chapel Hill classification of adult vasculitis.[2]

8.2 HENOCH–SCHÖNLEIN PURPURA (HSP)

8.2.1 Definition

This is a leucocytoclastic vasculitis, associated with immunoglobulin A deposition in the small vessels of skin and kidneys. Table 8.2 contains the proposed classification criteria.[1]

8.2.2 Epidemiology

This is the most common vasculitis in children, with an incidence of 14 per 100,000. It is more common in boys.

8.2.3 Etiology

Up to 80% of cases are preceded by an upper respiratory infection. Many organisms have been implicated, including streptococci.[3]

TABLE 8.1. New Classification of Childhood Vasculitis[1]

Predominantly large vessel vasculitis
  Takayasu arteritis

Predominantly medium-sized vessel vasculitis
  Childhood Polyarteritis Nodosa
  Cutaneous Polyarteritis
  Kawasaki Disease

Predominantly small vessel vasculitis
  Granulomatous
    Wegener granulomatosis
    Churg–Strauss syndrome
  Nongranulomatous
    Microscopic polyangiitis
    HSP
    Isolated cutaneous leucocytoclastic vasculitis
    Hypocomplementic urticarial vasculitis

Other vasculitides
  Behçet's disease
  Vasculitis secondary to infection (including Hepatitis B–associated
    PAN), malignancies and drugs, including hypersensitivity
    vasculitis
  Vasculitis associated with connective ı ssue diseases
  Isolated vasculitis of the central nervous system
  Cogan Syndrome
  Unclassified

TABLE 8.2. Classification Criteria for Henoch–Schönlein Purpura[1]

Palpable purpura (mandatory criterion) plus 1 of the following
criteria:
  Abdominal pain
  Any biopsy showing predominant IgA deposition
  Arthritis or arthralgia
  Renal involvement (any hematuria and/or proteinuria)

8.2.4 Clinical Manifestation

Children present with palpable purpura, typically occurring in the lower limbs (Figure 8.1), but can involve the upper limbs and face. Occasionally, the rash is edematous and can ulcerate. Common additional symptoms include arthralgia and arthritis (47 to 84%), and colicky abdominal pain (63 to 100%), which can be severe. Intussusception may occur in severe cases leading to

FIGURE 8.1. Palpable purpuric rash: Henoch–Schönlein Purpura.

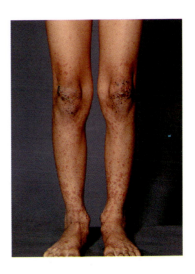

marked morbidity and mortality. Half have renal involvement (microscopic hematuria and mild proteinuria). Other symptoms include pulmonary involvement (most will have decreased diffusion capacity and, rarely, hemoptysis, or even pulmonary infarction), encephalopathy and orchitis.

8.2.5 Laboratory Findings
Platelet counts are normal or elevated, despite the purpura. There is a moderately raised white blood count and acute phase reactants. About half will have raised serum IgA.[4] Renal involvement is detectable as microscopic hematuria and proteinuria. In renal units, 5 to 10% is deemed severe enough for renal biopsy, which typically shows deposition of IgA in the mesangium. ANA and ANCA are negative.

8.2.6 Diagnosis
Palpable purpura, colicky abdominal pain and hematuria establish the diagnosis. A skin biopsy, if obtained, will show leucocytoclastic vasculitis with predominantly IgA deposition. Renal biopsy is recommended if there is significant proteinuria to exclude other causes and establish the presence of mesangial IgA immune complexes.

8.2.7 Treatment and Prognosis
The disease is, mostly, self-limiting so analgesia is often sufficient. Usually a mild disease with a monocylic course,

recurrences can occur over a few years. Nonsteroidal anti-inflammatory drugs are usually sufficient for symptomatic treatment of joint pain. Oral steroids are helpful for severe abdominal pain, necrotic skin rashes, heavy proteinuria and arthritis. Whether steroids alter the outcome of renal disease is controversial. Since approximately 20% of renal failures, presenting at the Great Ormond Street Hospital for Sick Children in London UK, are due to HSP, nephrologists there generally favour the use of steroids at 1 mg per kg per day for 14 days, or longer, as needed. Evidence-based protocols are needed.

8.3 LEUCOCYTOCLASTIC/HYPERSENSITIVITY VASCULITIS

8.3.1 Definition
This group is defined by the histological picture of leucocyte infiltration of the walls of small blood vessels. It is confined to the skin.

8.3.2 Epidemiology
Unknown.

8.3.3 Etiology
The causes are diverse, and there may be hypersensitivity reactions, for example, to drugs, or infection. It can also be idiopathic.

8.3.4 Clinical Manifestation
Leucocytoclastic vasculitis usually presents with a skin rash and no constitutional disturbances. The rash can be a fine, papular rash, or a red papular rash that looks like a blister and leaves a stain, or a bruise.

8.3.5 Laboratory Findings
Mildly increased ESR and C-reactive protein sometimes occurs, but no other laboratory abnormalities occur.

8.3.6 Diagnosis
Skin biopsy is the gold standard for diagnosis, as the histological appearances are typical.

8.3.7 Treatment and Prognosis
Treatment is symptomatic. A short course of steroids usually leads to complete recovery. Sometimes this is recurrent and a number of treatments have been favored anecdotally, including monthly IV immunoglobulin infusions, low doses of steroids and

colchicine. If the attacks are mild, no treatment is preferred, since the prognosis is benign.

8.4 HYPOCOMPLEMENTEMIC URTICARIAL VASCULITIS

8.4.1 Definition
Urticarial skin rash with the histological appearances of leucocytoclastic vasculitis on biopsy, associated with low serum complement levels.

8.4.2 Epidemiology
Unknown.

8.4.3 Etiology
Unknown.

8.4.4 Clinical Manifestations
Usually, a recurrent urticarial rash and lethargy. There are no other accompanying signs or symptoms.

8.4.5 Laboratory Findings
Low complement C4 and sometimes C3, a raised acute phase response with an elevated ESR and, occasionally, anemia of chronic disease.

8.4.6 Diagnosis
Apart from the above typical clinical and laboratory features it is important to exclude other causes, such as SLE, hypersensitivity reactions, cold or physically induced urticaria, by checking for antinuclear antibodies, double stranded DNA antibodies and a urine analysis. Finally, Chronic Infantile Neurologic Cutaneous Articular Syndrome (CINCA) can present, with a fixed urticarial rash and raised ESR, but there is usually an accompanying fever and the serum complement is normal.

8.4.7 Treatment and Prognosis
Treatment with a short course of oral steroids is effective. The condition may relapse, but the outcome is benign.

8.5 KAWASAKI DISEASE (KD)

8.5.1 Definition
This is a systemic vasculitis first described by Tomisaku Kawasaki in 1967, mainly affecting children under five years of age with high fevers, typical skin and mucous membrane involve-

TABLE 8.3. Classification Criteria for Kawasaki Disease[1]

Fever persisting for at least 5 days plus 4* of the following criteria:
Changes in peripheral extremities or perineal area
Polymorphous exanthema
Bilateral conjunctival injection
Changes of lips and oral cavity: Injection of oral and pharyngeal mucosa
Cervical Lymphadenopathy

*In the presence of coronary artery involvement detected on echocardiography and fever, fewer than 4 of the remaining 5 criteria are sufficient (exact number of criteria required to be defined in the validation phase).

ment and peeling of skin from extremities. The vessels involved are small and medium sized and, characteristically, produce coronary artery aneurysms. Table 8.3 contains the new proposed classification criteria for KD.[1]

8.5.2 Epidemiology
This is a systemic vasculitis, occurring most frequently in Japanese and Koreans between one and three years old. A Japanese survey of children under five from 1984 to 1994 reported an incidence of 94/100,000[5] and 6–10/100,000 has been reported in Caucasians under 5.[6] It is 1.5 times more common in boys.

8.5.3 Etiology
Often a history of a preceding infection. The fact that KD occurs as epidemics supports an infectious etiology. Activation of T lymphocytes, by superantigens from bacterial toxins, has been implicated as a cause.

8.5.4 Clinical Manifestations
High fevers for over one week, systemic disturbances, inflammation of the mucous membranes leading to conjunctival injection, red tongue, and lip ulcerations (Figure 8.2). Also, cervical lymphadenopathy and a nonspecific polymorphic skin rash. The child is highly irritable. Joint pains and arthritis are common. Features suggesting an upper respiratory tract infection, such as cough, coryza, and otitis media, as well as diarrhea, vomiting, ileus, jaundice, dysuria, pneumonitis, uveitis, convulsions and meningitis. Cardiac involvement includes myocarditis, pericarditis, tamponade and myocardial infarction.

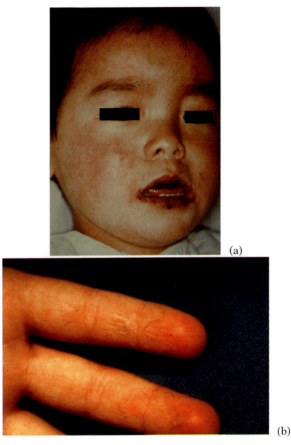

FIGURE 8.2. (a) KD showing facial rash and mucocutaneous ulcerations. (b) Peeling fingertips in KD.

8.5.5 Laboratory Findings

There is evidence of acute phase reaction with high ESR and CRP. Marked thrombocytosis often occurs as the fever resolves. Infection screen is negative, antinuclear antibodies are negative and serum complement is usually normal. Echocardiography shows coronary aneurysms (Figure 8.3) in over a quarter of untreated cases and may show myocarditis and pericaditis.

8.5.6 Diagnosis

Early diagnosis and treatment is essential, because of the risk of coronary artery aneurysms. Differential diagnoses include

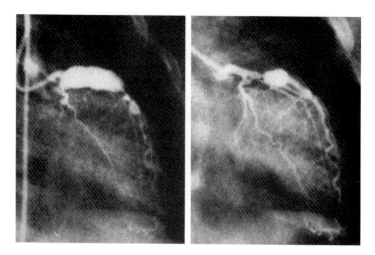

FIGURE 8.3. Coronary artery aneurysms on angiography.

infections, drug reactions, other rheumatological diseases, such as systemic JIA, reactive arthritis, and other vasculitides. An echocardiogram and ECG are essential if KD is suspected. Basic laboratory tests include FBC, platelet count, ESR, CRP, liver and renal function tests and urine analysis. "Incomplete" or "atypical" KD has been described by clinicians if five criteria are not met, but they could be other types of vasculitides (in particular polyarteritis nodosa) and a thorough search for alternative diagnoses is necessary.

8.5.7 Treatment

A child with suspected KD should be managed in hospital under a pediatrician. Symptomatic treatment consists of analgesia and rehydration. At onset, intravenous gammaglobulin (2 g/kg) should be given over 12 hours, followed by low dose aspirin (3–5 mg/kg/day). Sometimes the symptoms fail to respond, or return 24 hours after the first dose of immunoglobulin. In one reported series, 77% respond to treatment with IV immunoglobulin and 10 out of 15 patients in one series respond to retreatment.[7] Glucocorticoids are accepted as necessary at this stage and IV methylprednisolone (30 mg/kg), followed by oral prednisolone (1 mg/kg) should be continued until clinical signs of disease activity are abolished, before slow reduction. Oral aspirin should continue in order to prevent thrombotic events, as there is a high risk of such complication from inflammatory vessel damage, coupled with a high platelet count.

8.5.8 Outcome

The disease is monocyclic. The majority of patients with KD, without coronary aneurysms, recovered fully. Those children with coronary artery involvement have an increased risk of coronary heart disease in adult life[8] and will need long-term cardiac care.

8.6 POLYARTERITIS NODOSA (PAN) AND OTHER NECROTIZING VASCULITIDES

8.6.1 Definition

Polyarteritis nodosa is a systemic vasculitis characterized and defined by a typical histological appearance of necrotizing inflammatory changes in medium and/or smaller sized arteries. Table 8.4 contains the new proposed classification criteria for PAN.

8.6.2 Epidemiology

Polyarteritis nodosa is a rare vasculitis in childhood, with a mean age of onset of around nine years. The incidence appears equal in both sexes.[9,10]

8.6.3 Etiology

Childhood onset PAN can be a single acute episode following an infectious trigger, or a relapsing disease that has no obvious

TABLE 8.4. Classification Criteria for Childhood PAN[1]

The presence of at least 2 of the following criteria:
Skin involvement (livedo reticularis, tender subcutaneous nodules, other vasculitic lesions)
Myalgia or muscle tenderness
Systemic hypertension, relative to childhood normative data
Mononeuropathy or polyneuropathy
Abnormal urine analysis and/or impaired renal function
Testicular pain or tenderness
Signs or symptoms suggesting vasculitis of any other major organ system (gastrointestinal, cardiac, pulmonary, or central nervous system)
In the presence of (a mandatory criterion):
Biopsy showing small and midsize artery necrotizing vasculitis
Or
Angiographic abnormalities* (aneurysms or occlusions)

*Should include angiography if MRA is negative.

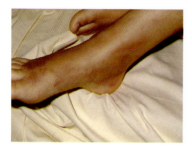

FIGURE 8.4. Livedo rash of polyarteritis nodosa.

infectious or other external triggers. It has been associated with streptococcal infection.[11,12]

8.6.4 Clinical Manifestation

PAN presents with fever of unknown origin, skin rash (palpable, painful and livedo reticularis [Figure 8.4]), lethargy, myalgia and weight loss. Arthralgia, abdominal pain and headaches are common. There is often evidence of renal involvement (e.g., proteinuria), neurological involvement, especially mononeuritis and, less commonly, cough/hemoptysis. In the European/Americas survey,[10] the skin, musculoskeletal and gastrointestinal systems were predominately involved. Renal and CNS involvement were also common.

Hepatitis B associated PAN (previously known as classical PAN) usually presents with fever, malaise, nephritic features, and orchitis. This is much rarer since the introduction of Hepatitis B vaccinations.

8.6.5 Laboratory Findings

All patients have raised acute phase reactants, anemia of chronic disease (hypochromic, microcytic anemia with normal ferritin). Cryoglobulins are characteristic of hepatitis B associated PAN. Disease specific autoantibodies, such as ANCA, should be absent. Other abnormal laboratory tests will depend on the affected organ system.

Skin and other organ biopsies show necrotizing vasculitis (Figure 8.5). Demonstration of aneurysms in medium-sized arteries, such as in the celiac trunk and renal arteries, are the diagnostic gold standard (Figure 8.6). MRA is often not sufficiently sensitive for the size of the vessels involved. Radioisotope imaging has been helpful in renal disease, when arteriograms were not readily available, showing attenuation of perfusion peripherally, as well as perfusion defects.

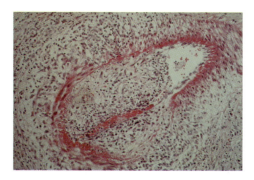

FIGURE 8.5. Histology of necrotizing vasculitis in polyarteritis nodosa.

8.6.6 Diagnosis

Any child with fever of unknown origin, irritability, myalgia, weight loss and unexplained multiple system involvement should have a vasculitis workup. This consists of exclusion of infectious cause of fever and other types of multisystem inflammatory diseases, such as SLE, microscopic polyangiitis, or Wegener's (see Sections 8.8 and 8.9). Diagnosis is supported by the

8

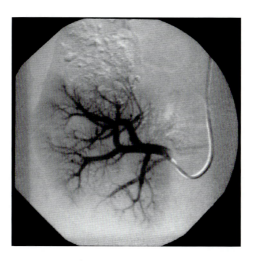

FIGURE 8.6. Aneurysms of the mesenteric arterial axis: Note that true aneurysms are seen along the vessel and not where there is increased contrast at the junction of vessel branches.

demonstration of raised ESR and CRP, along with abnormal tests for specific organ function and, ultimately, a biopsy, angiogram, or both.

8.6.7 Treatment

Pharmacological treatment consists of two phases, induction and maintenance. Induction is usually with IV methylprednisolone at 30 mg/kg and cyclophosphamide, given either as monthly pulses of 500 to 1000 mg/m^2 for 6 months, or orally for three months at 3 to 5 mg/kg. The cumulative dose of immunosuppressives remains a major concern. A cumulative dose of 200 to 250 mg/kg of cyclophosphamide is considered safe for most children, in terms of gonadal toxicity.[13] This would be roughly equal to three and a half months of oral cyclophosphamide at a dose of 2 mg/kg/day. Plasmapheresis and prostacylin/iloprost infusions, during the initiation stages of immunosuppression, are thought to be helpful to reduce vessel and tissue damage.

Azathioprine (2 to 3 mg/kg/day), or Colchicine at 1.5 to 2 mg/day, used in combination with low-dose steroid, are very effective in maintaining control after induction with steroids and cyclophosphamide.

One anti-TNF agent, infliximab, has proved encouraging and could be a good option for induction and/or maintenance. Anecdotally, anti-CD20 (rituximab) has proved helpful to control PAN, but further work needs to be undertaken before its recommendation. Finally, autologous stem cell transplant has been used in severe cases with some success.[14]

For hepatitis B associated disease, the treatment includes antiviral treatment and steroids.

8.6.8 Outcome

The course of PAN is variable depending on the organs involved. It is usually monocyclic, but can be relapsing, often with long periods of remission. The outcome, in the largest retrospective series[10] was much better than reported in adults with only one (1.1%) death and two (2.2%) with end stage renal disease. Similarly, recent pediatric series have all reported excellent results, much better than children treated before the establishment of treatment protocols in the 1990s.

8.7 CUTANEOUS POLYARTERITIS

Cutaneous polyarteritis is characterized by the presence of subcutaneous nodular, painful, nonpurpuric lesions with or without livedo reticularis and no systemic involvement, except for myalgia, arthralgia, and nonerosive arthritis. A deep skin biopsy that includes vessels in the subcutis, shows necrotizing non-granulomatous vasculitis. Tests for ANCA are negative. Cutaneous polyarteritis is often associated with serologic or microbiologic evidence of streptococcal infection and, by definition, does not include internal organ involvement. In the multicenter survey in Europe and the Americas, a majority had a preceding URTI.

8.7.1 Clinical Features

Rash is raised, red and painful with surrounding tissue edema. It occurs around the eyes and the instep of the foot (Figure 8.7). Rashes near the joint often cause periarticular edema and mimic arthritis by causing pain and restriction. The child is usually miserable and fractious, often with a history of a sore throat before the onset of rashes.

There have been reports of relapsing cutaneous polyarteritis, evolving into systemic PAN after penicillin prophylaxis was stopped.[12]

8.7.2 Laboratory Features

A marked acute phase response with increased markers of inflammation and microscopic anemia is seen. Urine analyses, renal and liver function tests are normal. Autoantibody screen is

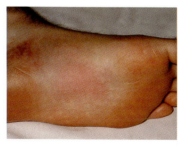

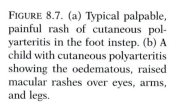

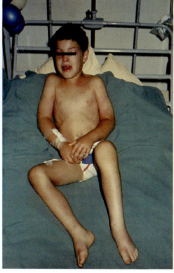

(a)

(b)

FIGURE 8.7. (a) Typical palpable, painful rash of cutaneous polyarteritis in the foot instep. (b) A child with cutaneous polyarteritis showing the oedematous, raised macular rashes over eyes, arms, and legs.

negative. Patients with poststreptococcal cutaneous PAN have very high titres of antistreptolysin O and anti-DNase B.

8.7.3 Diagnosis

A deep skin biopsy showing necrotizing vasculitis and the combination of the above clinical and laboratory features confirms diagnosis.

8.7.4 Treatment

Steroid therapy, in the form of pulse IV methylprednsolone at high doses (e.g., 30 mg/kg), followed by daily oral therapy at 1 mg/kg, aborts the inflammatory changes within 1 to 2 weeks. The steroid dose can then be tapered over the next few (up to 6) months. Relapses usually occur if this reduction is too fast, or alternate-day steroid dosages are used early in the disease course. Prophylactic penicillin should be given in cases where there is demonstrable recent streptococcal infection. Usually, the penicillin needs to be continued until postpuberty.

8.7.5 Outcome

The course of cutaneous polyarteritis is usually a benign one. The majority recover after a course of steroid therapy and a relapsing course suggests systemic involvement and a diagnosis of PAN.[12]

8.8 MICROSCOPIC POLYANGIITIS

This is a necrotizing pauci-immune vasculitis affecting small vessels and often associated with a high titer of Perinuclear Anti-Neutrophil Cytoplasmic Antibodies (p-ANCA), due to antibodies to Myeloperoxidase (MPO). Necrotizing glomerulonephritis is very common, as is pulmonary capillaritis without granulomatous lesions of the respiratory tract. The upper respiratory tract is spared.

8.8.1 Clinical Features

The presenting pulmonary symptoms are often acute, with pneumonia, hempotosis, fever and malaise. Pneumothoraces can occur. There is marked development of hypertension and nephritic features of proteinuria, hematuria, edema and renal failure.

8.8.2 Laboratory Features

Similar to PAN, but with the addition of a positive p-ANCA.

8.8.3 Diagnosis

A renal biopsy appearance of pauci-immune nephritis, together with the above clinical and laboratory features, clinch the diagnosis. The chest radiograph shows fluffy shadowing in the lung fields and, in the more severe cases, pneumothorax.

8.8.4 Treatment
Similar to PAN. Plasmapheresis, used concurrently with the induction therapy, improves the prognosis of microscopic PAN.

8.8.5 Outcome
Mortality is high with pulmonary involvement. End stage renal disease can occur.

8.9 WEGENER'S GRANULOMATOSIS (WG)

8.9.1 Definition
This is a granulomatous vasculitis, mainly affecting the upper and lower respiratory and renal tracts. Table 8.5 shows the new proposed classification criteria for WG.[1]

8.9.2 Epidemiology
It is rare in children and constitutes 1.4% and 2.2% of the pediatric rheumatic diseases in the USA and Canadian registries, respectively.

8.9.3 Etiology
Unknown.

8

8.9.4 Clinical Manifestation
Patients often present with fever, malaise, weight loss and, occasionally, "pseudotumor of the orbit." More specifically, they present with chronic painful sinusitis, otitis, or pneumonia unresponsive to antibiotics. Other symptoms include hoarse voice, cough, dyspnoea, hearing loss and hemoptysis. Collapse of the nasal bridge is a common sign (Figure 8.8). Hematuria, with or without hypertension, indicates renal involvement. Arthralgia

TABLE 8.5. Classification Criteria for Wegener's Granulomatosis[1]

The presence of 3 of the following criteria:
Abnormal urinalysis*
Granulomatous inflammation on biopsy
Nasal–sinus inflammation
Subglottic, tracheal, or endobronchial stenosis
Abnormal chest X-ray or CT
PR3-ANCA or C-ANCA staining

*If kidney biopsy is performed, it characteristically shows necrotizing pauci-immune glomerulonephritis.

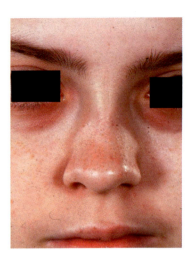

FIGURE 8.8. Typical saddle-shaped nose of Wegener granulomatosis.

and arthritis are common. There can be a nodular skin rash and deep oral and nasal ulceration.

8.9.5 Laboratory Findings

There is evidence of acute phase response, as in all vasculitides. In addition, antineutrophil cytoplasmic antibodies are frequently present in the serum, with a cytosolic pattern (c-ANCA), mainly directed against proteinase 3 (PR3).

Tomography, or CT of the glottis and subglottis, show inflammatory infiltration and narrowing of the airways, which frequently leads to collapse of the airways during inspiration (Figure 8.9a). Subglottic stenosis is more frequent in children than adults. Chest radiographs often show multifocal shadows (Figure 8.9b), and, occasionally, the classical cavitating lesion that is often seen in adults. Typically, the histology of the lesions shows a necrotizing vasculitis with granulomata.

8.9.6 Diagnosis

Upper respiratory tract CT images are characteristic and biopsies are diagnostic. Involvement of the subglottis and larger bronchi are typical. High titre c-ANCA, due to anti-PR3, is diagnostic. These tests would differentiate WG from microscopic polyangiitis in particular, as the latter is nongranulomatous and is positive p-ANCA (anti-MPO). Limited WG can exist without renal lesions.

8.9.7 Treatment

Induction treatment is similar to PAN. Regarding the newer biologics, infliximab is effective, but not etanercept. There has been

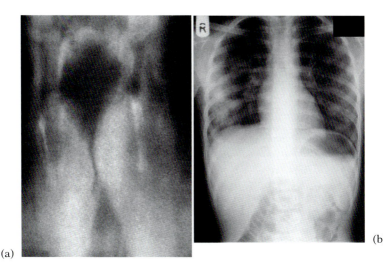

(a)

(b)

FIGURE 8.9. (a) Tomogram showing narrowing of the glottis by granulomatous tissue. (b) Chest x-ray of a child with Wegener granulomatosis.

an association of disease flares with staphylocci infections, so treatment with trimethoprin/sulphamethoxazole is often added. During the maintenance phase of the disease, methotrexate (up to 20 mg/kg/day), or azathioprine, are often effective. Treatment is for life, as relapses invariably occur on withdrawal of treatment.

8.9.8 Outcome
This is a relapsing disease that requires regular reviews by a rheumatologist, otolaryngologist and nephrologist throughout life.

8.10 BEHÇET'S DISEASE (BD)

8.10.1 Definition
A systemic vasculitis, with characteristic oral and genital ulcers, vasculopathy and uveitis.

8.10.2 Epidemiology
Behçet's disease is more common in certain ethnic groups around the Mediterranean (such as Cypriots, Greeks, Turks) and the Japanese and is familial in these populations. It usually presents in the second and third decade and is rare in children

(prevalence <1 : 15,000 in Turks). It is sporadic in North America and frequently lacks uveitis.

8.10.3 Etiology
HLA B51 has been found to be associated with Turkish families with BD, but the etiology remains unclear.

8.10.4 Clinical Manifestations
The oral ulcerations are often multiple, deep and painful, affecting unusual areas (such as the tongue and throat), as well as usual sites seen with apthous ulceration. Scarring can occur with deep ulcerations of the oral and genital areas. The vasculitis affects both the arterial and venous systems and thrombotic venous and arterial events are classical signs of this disease, which can be clearly seen in the retina. Skin rashes can vary from nodular lesions, like erythema nodosum, to a leucocytoclastic lesion. There is often a history of papular reaction to a needle prick, the pathergy phenomenon. The latter is more common in the Mediterranean racial groups. The patient can present with colitis. The skin, eye, the CNS and GI tracts are most frequently affected. Arthralgia and arthritis are common.

8.10.5 Laboratory Findings
No specific tests. The laboratory findings are those of a vasculitis with increased acute phase response.

8.10.6 Diagnosis
The criteria, proposed by an international study group in 1990, requires the presence of recurrent oral ulceration, plus two of the following:

- recurrent genital ulceration
- eye lesions (typical posterior uveitis, with thrombotic features in arteries and veins)
- skin lesions (nodular/purpura/ulcers/folliculitis)
- positive pathergy test (often indicated by a history of skin lesions at sites of needle entry in blood tests)

In addition to the above, a survey by history, examination and appropriate imaging and laboratory tests is important to define the extent of organ involvement and exclude other rheumatic and infectious diseases.

8.10.7 Treatment

No controlled studies have been performed in children with BD. Adult studies have shown that for mucocutaneous BD, Colchicine (up to 1.5 mg/day) was effective, as was thalidomide. These have been used with effect in children. For more severe ulcerations, steroids are helpful. Low-dose steroids, in combination with thalidomide (2.5 mg/kg/dy), have been effective in Caucasian children. A combination of the three drugs has been used as maintenance. In severe vasculitis with uveitis and organ involvement, pulse IV methylprednisolone and cyclophosphamide have been used. Azathioprine (1 mg/kg) and Cyclosporin A (3 to 5 mg/kg) may help with retinal disease. Anti-TNF agents have been helpful. Table 8.6 illustrates the treatment algorithm for Behçet's disease used at Great Ormond Street Hospital, London, UK.

8.10.8 Outcome

Disease intensity usually abates over time, however, Behçet's disease is a significant cause of mortality, especially due to

TABLE 8.6. Treatment Algorithm for Behçet's Disease

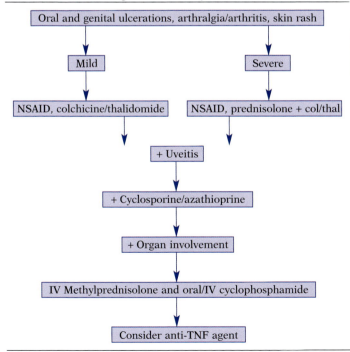

bleeding pulmonary artery aneurysms, among young male patients. Uveitis can be a significant cause of blindness.[15]

Other causes of mortality are ruptured peripheral aneurysms, severe central nervous system disease, Budd–Chiari Syndrome and intestinal ulceration and perforation, which is especially prominent among the Japanese.

References

1. Ozen S, Ruperto N, Dillon MJ et al. EULAR/PReS endorsed consensus criteria for the classification of childhood vasculitides. *Ann Rheum Dis*. 2006;65:936–941.
2. Jennette JC, Falk RJ, Andrassy K et al. Nomenclature of systemic vasculitides. Proposal of an international consensus conference. *Arthritis Rheum*. 1994;37:187–192.
3. Bagga A, Dillon MJ. Leukocytoclastic Vasculitis, in *Textbook for Paediatric Rheumatology*, 4th ed. Cassidy JT, Petty RE, eds., Philadelphia: W.B. Saunders Company; 2001:569–579.
4. White RHR. Henoch-Schönlein purpura. In: Churg A, Churg J, eds. *Systemic Vasculitides*. New York: Igaku-Shoin Medical Publishers; 1991:203–217.
5. Yashiro M, Nakamura Y, Hirose K et al. Surveillance of Kawasaki disease in Japan, 1985–1994. In: Kato H. ed. *Kawasaki Disease*. Amsterdam: Elsevier Science; 1995:15–21.
6. Barron KS, Shulman ST, Rowley A et al. Report of the National Institutes of Health Workshop on Kawasaki Disease. *J Rheumatol*. 1999;26:170–190.
7. Wallace CA, French JW, Kahn SJ et al. Initial intravenous gammaglobulin treatment failure in Kawasaki disease. *Pediatrics*. 2000; 105:E78.
8. Iemura M, Ishii M, Sugimura T et al. Long term consequences of regressed coronary aneurysms after Kawasaki disease: vascular wall morphology and function. *Heart*. 2000;83:307–311.
9. Dillon MJ. Childhood vasculitis. *Lupus*. 1998;7:259–265.
10. Ozen S, Anton J, Arisoy N et al. Juvenile polyarteritis: results of a multicenter survey of 110 children. *J Pediatr*. 2004;145:517–522.
11. Albornoz MA, Benedetto AV, Korman M et al. Relapsing cutaneous polyarteritis nodosa associated with streptococcal infections. *Int J Dermatol*. 1998;37:664–666.
12. David J, Ansell BM, Woo P. Polyarteritis nodosa associated with streptococcus. *Arch Dis Child*. 1993;69:685–688.
13. Latta K, von Schnakenburg C, Ehrich JH. A meta-analysis of cytotoxic treatment for frequently relapsing nephrotic syndrome in children. *Pediatr Nephrol*. 2001;16:271–282.
14. Wedderburn LR, Jeffery R, White H et al. Autologous stem cell transplantation for paediatric-onset polyarteritis nodosa: changes in autoimmune phenotype in the context of reduced diversity of the T- and B-cell repertoires, and evidence for reversion from the

CD45RO(+) to RA(+) phenotype. *Rheumatology (Oxford)*. 2001; 40:1299–1307.

15. Yazici H, Basaran G, Hamuryudan V et al. The ten-year mortality in Behcet's syndrome. *Br J Rheumatol.* 1996;35:139–141.

Chapter 9
Lyme Arthritis

9.1 INTRODUCTION

Steere et al. discovered Lyme disease in the 1970's while investigating an outbreak of childhood arthritis in Old Lyme, Connecticut.[1] It was subsequently found to be due to a tick borne spirochete, *Borrelia burgdorferi*.

9.2 DEFINITION

Lyme disease is characterised by a flu-like illness followed by cutaneous disease (erythema migrans), and then, in some, neurologic (Bell's Palsy, meningitis, radiculoneuropathy, and encephalopathy), cardiac (heart block and congestive heart failure) or arthritis; all due to *B. burgdorferi*.[2]

9.3 EPIDEMIOLOGY

Lyme arthritis is limited to the Northern Hemisphere in temperate regions where the vector is found, generally in central Europe (although it is described throughout the entire European continent) and in North America, especially in in the northeastern United States and northern Midwest. It is rare in Asia. It occurs equally in boys and girls and has been reported in children of all ages, especially in those exposed to ticks (children who play in the woods and young adults who hike or camp).

9.4 ETIOLOGY

Lyme disease results from an infection with the spirochete *B. burgdorferi* that is transmitted by an Ixodes tick. This is a very small tick, not the wood tick more frequently found on pets. The primary reservoir for the organism is white-footed mice, voles, and deer; humans are incidental hosts.

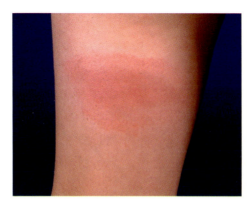

FIGURE 9.1. Typical erythema migrans showing the expanding target lesion. (Courtesy of Lawrence Zemel, MD.)

9.5 CLINICAL MANIFESTATIONS

The tick prefers to feed in warm moist areas so the bite usually occurs in the groin, axilla, breast, and neck. It is at this site, 1 to 2 weeks later, that the initial rash will develop. It is a painless enlarging annular lesion that clears centrally as it enlarges peripherally giving it a ring-like appearance, known as erythema migrans (Figure 9.1). Flu-like symptoms may accompany the rash. The next most common manifestation is arthritis that will follow the rash by weeks to months and is typically a monarthritis of the knee with massive swelling, frequently without pain. The arthritis lasts a few days or weeks and completely resolves, but may recur months later. About a third of the patients with arthritis have an oligoarthritis pattern of joint involvement and only rarely is it polyarticular. Other, less common features are Bell's palsy, encephalitis, uveitis, carditis, and heart block. Neurological involvement in Lyme can occur, but not in the absence of prior characteristic Lyme disease.[2]

9.6 LABORATORY FEATURES

The IgM antibody response to the Lyme spirochete peaks 2 to 6 weeks after infection and disappears within another month. The IgM peak is followed by prolonged IgG antibody production. Initially, screening for both IgM and IgG done by enzyme immunosorbent assay (EIA) or immunofluorescence assay IFA for these antibodies should be obtained. However, these are fraught with false positives so all positive or equivocal tests should be confirmed with Western Blot testing for specific antibody production again different spirochetal outer surface proteins (Osp). IgM antibodies against 2 of 3 Osp are confirmatory of recent infection; most of these children will also have positive IgG antibodies to 5 of 10 Osp bands. Virtually all patients have an antibody response to the spirochete.[3] The ANA and RF tests are negative.

Synovial fluid is inflammatory with an average of 25,000 white blood cells per cm[3].[4] PCR of the synovial fluid may help in isolated patients in whom the diagnosis is not readily apparent, although it generally is not needed.

9.7 ESTABLISHING THE DIAGNOSIS

The diagnosis of Lyme arthritis is generally straightforward, even if there is no history of tick bite and rash but reasonable temporal and geographic exposure to the tick. The joint is massively swollen with little pain. The synovial fluid is inflammatory. Testing for both IgG and IgM antibodies reveal a positive screen by EIA or IFA and is confirmed by Western blot testing with at least 2 of 3 IgM positive bands and 5 of 10 IgG positive bands.[2,3]

9.8 TREATMENT

Lyme arthritis is usually successfully treated with doxycycline 100 mg orally twice daily for 2 to 4 weeks, or amoxicillin 500 mg or 17 mg/kg TID for 3 to 4 weeks in children less than 9 years of age or in pregnant women since doxycycline will stain enamel in the forming tooth.[5] Cefuroxime axetil is a better alternative for the penicillin allergic, the macrolides (including erythromycin and azithromycin) being less effective clinically. Occasionally, intravenous cefuroxime may be necessary if the initial treatment fails. Jarisch–Herxheimer-like reactions may occur after starting therapy, mostly manifest by fever and arthralgias. See Table 9.1 for alternatives and courses depending on disease manifestations.

Intra-articular corticosteroids given prior to antibiotic treatment have been implicated in a more chronic arthritis, but have also been associated with decreasing the duration of synovitis if given after the course of antibiotics.[6]

9.9 OUTCOME

Lyme disease has an excellent prognosis.[7] The vast majority of features are self-limited. Children with Lyme arthritis generally do very well with either the initial course of oral antibiotics or, if needed, an intravenous course (with or without an intraarticular injection of corticosteroids). If the arthritis does not resolve, then the diagnosis needs to be reconsidered.[8] The anxiety

TABLE 9.1. Treatment Regimens for Lyme Disease

Agents (mg given per dose)
  Doxycycline 100 mg PO BID (over age 8 years)
  Amoxicillin 500 or 17 mg/kg PO TID (under age 8 years or
    pregnant)
  Cefuroxime axetil 500 mg or 15 mg/kg PO BID
  Erythromycin 500 mg or 12.5 mg/kg PO QID (less effective)
  Azithromycin 500 mg or 10 mg/kg PO (less effective)
  Clarithromycin 500 Mg or 7.5 mg/kg PO BID (less effective)
  Penicillin G 4 million units or 50,000 units/kg IV every 4 hours
  Ceftriaxone sodium 2 g or 75–100 mg/kg IV single daily dose
  Cefotaxime sodium 2 g or 50 mg/kg IV every 8 hours
  Chloramphenicol 1 g or 12.5 mg/kg IV every 6 hours

Erythema migrans
  Doxycycline, amoxicillin, cefuroxime axetil, erythromycin,
    azithromycin or clarithromycin PO for 14–21 days (7 days for
    azithromycin).

Lyme arthritis
  Doxycycline or amoxicillin PO for 21–28 days
  If fails: Ceftriaxone sodium or Penicillin G IV for 30 days

Bell's palsy
  Doxycycline or amoxicillin PO for 21–28 days

Central Nervous System Lyme
  Ceftriaxone sodium or penicillin G IV for 30 days
  Alternatives: Cefotaxime sodium or chloramphenicol IV for 30 days

Carditis
  Mild: Doxycycline or amoxicillin PO for 14–21 days
  Severe: Ceftriaxone sodium or penicillin G IV for 14–21 days

surrounding the mythical "Chronic Lyme disease" needs to be directly and compassionately dealt with early on to prevent unnecessary disability and prolonged courses of antibiotics.[9]

References

1. Steere AC, Malawista SE, Snydrian DR et al. Lyme arthritis: an epidemic of oligoarticular arthritis in children and adults in three connecticut communities. *Arthritis Rheum*. 1977;20:7–17.
2. Stanek G, Strle F. Lyme borreliosis. *Lancet*. 2003;362:1639–1647.
3. DePietropaolo DL, Powers JH, Gill JM et al. Diagnosis of lyme disease. *Am Fam Physician*. 2005;72:297–304.
4. Eichenfield AH, Goldsmith DP, Bench JL et al. Childhood Lyme arthritis: experience in an endemic area. *J Pediatr*. 1986;109:753–758.

5. *Lyme Disease (Borrelia burgdorferi Infection)*. In *Red Book: 2003 Report of the Committee on Infectious Diseases*. Pickering L, Ed., American Academy of Pediatrics 2003;407–411.
6. Bentas W, Karch H, Huppertz HI. Lyme arthritis in children and adolescents: outcome 12 months after initiation of antibiotic therapy. *J Rheumatol*. 2000;27:2025–2030.
7. Huppertz HI, Karch H, Suschke HJ et al. Lyme arthritis in European children and adolescents. The Pediatric Rheumatology Collaborative Group. *Arthritis Rheum*. 1995;38:361–368.
8. Sood SK, Rubin LG, Blades ME et al. Positive serology for Lyme borreliosis in patients with juvenile rheumatoid arthritis in a Lyme borreliosis endemic area: analysis by immunoblot. *J Rheumatol*. 1993;20:739–741.
9. Sigal LH, Hassett AL. Contributions of societal and geographical environments to "chronic Lyme disease": the psychopathogenesis and aporology of a new "medically unexplained symptoms" syndrome. *Environ Health Perspect*. 2002;4:607–611.

Chapter 10
Autoinflammatory Syndromes

10.1 INTRODUCTION

Fever in a child usually indicates an infection. When the fever is prolonged or recurrent, the differential diagnosis widens to include more occult infections, inflammatory bowel disease; autoimmune diseases, systemic vasculitides, malignancy, or one group of diseases in which fever plays a prominent role. This group is characterized by periodic recurrences, positive family history and characteristic clinical features, and are called autoinflammatory syndromes.[1] Typically, the children will be entirely well in between attacks and have normal growth rates despite repeated disruptions to their health and routines. These diseases are also known as "recurrent fever syndromes" (Table 10.1). Systemic onset juvenile idiopathic arthritis (JIA) might be included as an autoinflammatory syndrome, as discussed elsewhere in this book (see Chapter 3). Summaries of the clinical and genetic aspects of the autoinflammatory syndromes are in Tables 10.2 and 10.3.

10.2 FAMILIAL MEDITERRANEAN FEVER (FMF)

10

FMF was the first recurrent fever to be recognized to have a genetic basis and is marked by its early age of onset, serious morbidity and potential mortality if not treated adequately.

10.2.1 Etiology

FMF is an autosomal recessive disease, due to a mutation of the MEFV gene, on the short arm of chromosome 12, that codes for a protein called "pyrin" or "marenostrin."[2] This gene is expressed primarily in granulocytes and the protein is thought to reduce inflammation. Abnormalities in the protein may allow inflammation to proceed unabated. At least 25 distinct mutations in MEFV have been identified and they seem to correlate with disease severity, course, and outcome. The most common

TABLE 10.1. The Autoinflammatory Syndromes

Familial Mediterranean Fever
Hyperimmunoglobulinemia D and Autoinflammatory Syndromes
Tumor Necrosis Factor Associated Periodic Syndrome
Familial Cold Autoinflammatory Syndrome
Muckle–Well Syndrome
Chronic Infantile Neurological Cutaneous and Articular Syndrome
Periodic Fever, Aphthous Stomatitis, Pharyngitis, and Adenopathy
   Syndrome
Systemic Juvenile Idiopathic Arthritis

mutation is a substitution of methionine for valine at position 694 (M694V). Mutations in MEFV may play a role in other disorders marked by inflammation, including PFAPA.

10.2.2 Epidemiology

FMF affects mainly populations of Mediterranean origin. Other populations are less frequently affected. The majority of patients experience their first attack before the age of 10 years, and roughly 20% experience it before 2 years of age. Males and females are affected equally.

10.2.3 Clinical Features

FMF is characterized by frequent, recurrent high fever, lasting for one to three days and accompanied by serosal inflammation (pleuritis, peritonitis, and synovitis). The peritonitis may mimic an acute surgical abdomen. The fever is of rapid onset, 38 to 40°C (100 to 104°F) and early on can be the only manifestation. Intervals between attacks vary from weeks to months and may be triggered by stress, infection and trauma. Patients are well between attacks, but may have high laboratory markers of inflammation. Peritonitis occurs in 95% of patients, but not necessarily with each attack and is more often accompanied by diarrhea than constipation. Pleuritis occurs in 25 to 80% of patients and is associated with typical pleuritic chest pain. Arthritis occurs in 25 to 75% of patients, commonly presenting as an acute large joint mono- or oligoarthritis. Rarely, a destructive arthritis occurs and can include the sacroiliac joints. The symptoms can be so severe with swelling, redness, heat and pain that FMF may be confused with septic arthritis. Erysipelas-like skin lesions, primarily on the lower extremities, can accompany attacks and usually resolve over

TABLE 10.2. Clinical Autoinflammatory Syndromes

	FMF	HIDS	TRAPS	MWS	FCAS	CINCA	P-FAPA
Age of onset	Majority <5 years	Within first year	Any	Within first year	Within first year	Neonatal	Majority <5 years
Duration of attacks	1–3 days	3–7 days	>7 days	2–3 days	12–24 hours	Long-lasting	3–6 days
Skin	Erysipelas-like lesions	Maculopapular, urticarial	Plaques; painful, migratory	Urticaria	Cold-induced urticaria	Urticaria	Unaffected
MSK	Monoarthritis, myalgias	Arthralgias, occasionally oligoarthritis	Myalgia	Arthralgia	Arthralgia	Irregular ossification, epiphyseal overgrowth, destructive arthritis	Arthralgias occasionally
Abdominal/ GI	Peritonitis splenomegaly	Abdominal pain	Abdominal pain	Occasional pain	Nausea	Hepatosplenomegaly	Abdominal pain rarely
Ocular	Rare	Rare	Conjunctivitis, periorbital edema	Conjunctivitis, episcleritis	Occasional conjunctivitis	Papilledema, conjunctivitis, uveitis, blindness	Unaffected

TABLE 10.2. *Continued*

	FMF	HIDS	TRAPS	MWS	FCAS	CINCA	P-FAPA
Other features	Scrotal swelling, vasculitis	Cervical lymphadenopathy, oral ulcers	Inguinal hernia	Sensorineural hearing loss	Rigors	Sensorineural hearing loss, developmental and growth delay, chronic meningitis, raised intracranial pressure, frontal bossing	Tonsillitis, oral ulcers, cervical lymphadenopathy
Amyloidosis	Yes	One case reported	Yes	Yes	Yes	Yes	No
Treatment	Colchicine	Etanercept/anakinra	Etanercept	Anakinra	Stanozolol, anakinra	Anakinra	Short course of corticosteroids, prophylactic cimetidine or tonsillectomy

TABLE 10.3. Genetics of Autoinflammatory Syndromes

	FMF	HIDS	TRAPS	MWS	FCAS	CINCA	P-FAPA
Inheritance	AR	AR, or sporadic	AD	AD	AD	AD, or sporadic	Unknown
Chromosome	16p13	12q24	12p13	1q44	1q44	1q44	Unknown
Gene	MEFV	MVK	TNFRSF1A	CIAS1	CIAS1	CIAS1	Unknown
Protein	Pyrin (marenostrin)	Mevalonate kinase	Tumor necrosis factor receptor 1	Cryopyrin	Cryopyrin	Cryopyrin	Unknown

AR = autosomal recessive; AD = autosomal dominant

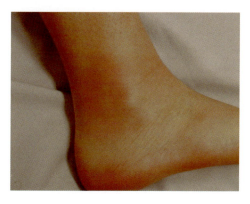

FIGURE 10.1. Erisypelas-like erythema overlying the right lateral malleolus in a 14-year-old girl with FMF. (Courtesy of Dr. Shai Padeh.)

2 to 3 days (Figure 10.1). Other manifestations include myalgia, orchitis and splenomegaly. Patients from certain ethnic groups (e.g., North African, Jews, and Turks) are more likely to develop familial amyloidosis. The disease course seems to correlate with the genotype, with the most severe courses being associated with patients who are homozygous for the M694V genotype.

10.2.4 Laboratory Features and Diagnosis

The diagnosis of FMF is based on the characteristic clinical manifestations, response to colchicine and family history. Criteria have been proposed, which have a very high sensitivity and specificity for the diagnosis of FMF. The diagnosis can be supported by genetic testing, but not all patients that fulfill the criteria have mutations of pyrin, suggesting that there are mutations yet to be identified. Therefore, the diagnosis remains clinical. Laboratory changes include elevated acute phase reactants during the attacks, which may not return to normal between attacks.

10.2.5 Treatment

Colchicine is the treatment of choice.[3] It reduces the frequency and severity of attacks and prevents the development of amyloidosis. However, there may only be a partial response in some cases, even with good adherence. NSAIDs may be effective in the treatment of arthritis. Since it is not possible to predict who will develop amyloidosis and who will be spared, colchicine use should be life long, even in the absence of symptoms. The dose of colchicine used is 0.5 to 2 mg per day, usually in divided doses. The major side effects are abdominal pain and diarrhea. It is safe to use colchicine during pregnancy and also for prolonged periods (i.e., many years).

10.2.6 Outcome
The use of colchicine has dramatically improved the outcome of patients with FMF, 50% of whom eventually developed amyloidosis.

10.3 PERIODIC FEVER, APHTHOUS STOMATITIS, PHARYNGITIS, AND ADENOPATHY (PFAPA) SYNDROME
PFAPA Syndrome is probably one of the more common autoinflammatory fevers syndromes in non-Mediterranean populations. It is marked by recurrences of attacks every 2 to 8 weeks, starting in early life (usually 2 to 4 years of age).[4] Attacks consist of abrupt fever spikes, generalized malaise, tonsillitis (no pathogens identified) and tender cervical lymphadenopathy. Painful oral ulcers are common during attacks, but not all features develop consistently with each attack. The outcome is good and most patients generally "outgrow" the disease during their second decade. Corticosteroids given at the onset of attacks for 1 to 2 days are very effective. Other treatments have included prophylactic cimetidine, antibiotics and tonsillectomy. No genetic defects have been consistently identified to date.

10.4 HYPERIMMUNOGLOBULINEMIA D SYNDROME (HIDS)
HIDS was originally described by a group of Dutch patients almost 20 years ago. It is marked by recurrent attacks of fever and systemic inflammation, beginning very early in life, in association with elevated levels of serum IgD.[5] The high IgD levels are not specific to HIDS and are occasionally seen in FMF and PFAPA.

10.4.1 Etiology
HIDS is a rare autosomal recessive disease, with approximately 200 cases described to date. One of the susceptibility genes for HIDS codes for mevalonate kinase (MVK), which is located on the short arm of chromosome 12 and is responsible for catalyzing the metabolism of mevalonate in the isoprenoid biosynthesis pathway. Severe reductions in enzyme activity (<5% activity) result in the disease mevalonic aciduria and 5 to 15% acitivity is found in HIDS. How the metabolic defect leads to bouts of severe repeated inflammation is not yet understood.

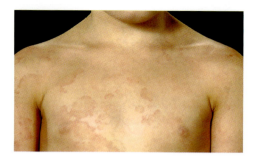

FIGURE 10.2. The HIDs rash is typically over the whole body, including the palms of the hand. It is often described as erythema marginatum and is fixed.

10.4.2 Epidemiology

HIDS usually starts within the first year of life. Most affected patients described so far are of Dutch or French origin. Males and females are affected equally.

10.4.3 Clinical Features

The attacks of fever are somewhat longer in duration compared to FMF, lasting 2 to 7 days, with an irregular periodicity, anywhere from once every 2 weeks to every several months. Fever rises abruptly, often with chills and climbs quickly up to 40°C (104°F). Usually, there is no precipitant, but trauma, illness, and, in particular, immunization may initiate an attack. Prominent symptoms during attacks are gastrointestinal (nausea, vomiting, diarrhea, abdominal pain). Other symptoms are arthralgia, lower limb oligoarthritis, and tender cervical lymphadenopathy, often unilateral. Splenomegaly and hepatomegaly are common in children, but rare in adults. A variety of rashes, including macular, papular, maculopapular, urticarial, nodular purpuric, and erythema marginatum, on the trunk, limbs, and palms are frequent with attacks (Figure 10.2), as are oral apthous ulcers. Attacks tend to lessen in frequency with age.

10.4.4 Laboratory Features and Diagnosis

The typical clinical pattern, together with a raised serum IgD and the presence of MVK mutation provide the diagnosis. However, some typical patients have normal IgD levels, and elevated IgD levels may be found in patients with other diseases. Elevated levels of serum IgA often accompany the high IgD levels. Raised acute phase reactants are seen during the attacks, but return to normal values in between. Most patients have heterozygous mutations in the MVK gene, with V377I being the most common. Urinary mevalonic acid may be mildly elevated during an attack of HIDS.

10.4.5 Treatment
Recent case reports show that treatment with etanercept is effective,[6] in addition to anecdotal reports of benefit with anakinra, colchicine, corticosteroids, intravenous immunoglobulin, and cyclosporine. Usually, there is a typical history of initial improvements followed by a return to the previous recurrent patterns, with the possible exception of etanercept and anakinra.

10.4.6 Outcome
The frequency and severity of attacks lessen with age. Fortunately, long-term sequelae are rare. To date these have included peritoneal adhesions and crescentic glomerulonephritis, and amyloidosis.

10.5 TUMOR NECROSIS FACTOR-RECEPTOR-ASSOCIATED PERIODIC SYNDROME (TRAPS)
TRAPS was originally described in a large Irish family cohort and so was called familial hibernian fever. The genetic basis for this syndrome, a mutation in the gene encoding the TNF p55 receptor, has allowed for the inclusion of other families.[7]

10.5.1 Etiology
TRAPS is due to a mutation of the TNFRSF1A gene on the short arm of chromosome 12, responsible for coding the type I TNF receptor (or CD120a). Mutations alter the structure of the 2 extracellular domains of TNFSFR1A. The normal receptor transduces the signal of TNF-α, but is also shed from the cell surface as soluble receptor, capable of binding free TNF and, thus, preventing cellular stimulation. The mutation reduces shedding of the receptor, allowing continuous cellular stimulation and maintenance of the inflammatory response.

10.5.2 Epidemiology
TRAPS is an autosomal dominant disorder, but sporadic cases do occur. It has been reported most frequently in families with Celtic origins in Ireland and Great Britain, but the disease is being identified more regularly in patients from other

backgrounds. Most patients have their onset in childhood, but symptoms may be delayed until mid-adulthood. Males and females are equally affected.

10.5.3 Clinical Features

Attacks may be short lived, but tend to be much longer in duration compared to HIDS or FMF and, occasionally, last several weeks. They are accompanied by myalgias, which are often migratory. Macular skin rashes and plaques are common, and may be painful (Figure 10.3). Ocular features, conjunctivitis and periorbital edema help differentiate TRAPS from other autoinflammatory syndromes. Other clinical features include colicky abdominal pain, diarrhea or constipation arthralgia of large joints (rarely arthritis), inguinal hernia, testicular pain and pleuritic chest pain. Occasionally, memory loss, or lack of concentration, have been described. The attacks may be precipitated by stress, illness and vigorous exercise. Amyloidosis may develop in up to 25% of patients.

10.5.4 Laboratory Features and Diagnosis

During attacks, laboratory tests reflect signs of acute inflammation, with elevated acute phase reactants. The diagnosis is made in the face of typical presentation and a positive family history.

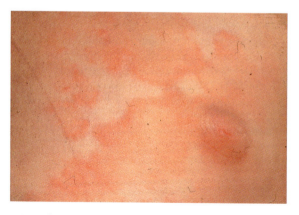

FIGURE 10.3. This TRAPs rash was from a boy with familial TRAPS. Its location is on the leg. It is present during attacks, but can be absent in between.

10.5.5 Treatment

Attacks may be ameliorated by NSAIDs but dramatically reduced by prednisone. The dose required to prevent attacks will lead to toxicity and alternative treatments are needed. Soluble TNF receptor in the form of subcutaneous etanercept twice weekly has proven most beneficial.[7] The exact dosing regime has not yet been established.

10.5.6 Outcome

Attacks, although irregular, are lifelong. Amyloidosis develops in approximately 25% of patients.

10.6 THE CIAS1 SYNDROMES

The following three syndromes are all characterized by autosomal dominant transmission (although sporadic cases do occur), early age of onset and mutations in a gene, which goes by several terms, including NALP3, CIAS1 and PYPAF1. This gene is located on chromosome 1 and encodes a 105 kDa protein called cryopyrin. Cryopyrin, like pyrin, is expressed in granulocytes as well as monocytes and chondrocytes. Interestingly, a single mutation in different parts of the CIAS1 can result in different diseases and the observed clinical spectrum in each individual disease suggests that other factors play a role in determining the phenotypic expression of the mutation.[8] They range in a spectrum of severity. Recent advances suggest that this gene is involved in the processing of interleukin-1β, and, therefore, treatment of these diseases with interleukin-1 blockade-anakinra, is effective in aborting attacks and preventing long-term complications.

10.7 FAMILIAL COLD AUTOINFLAMMATORY SYNDROME (FCAS)

This syndrome usually begins very early in infancy and is transmitted in an autosomal dominant pattern with complete penetrance. Attacks are precipitated 2 to 3 hours after cold exposure and consist of high fever, rashes and arthralgias, conjunctivitis, headaches, myalgia and fatigue. Urticarial lesions may start distally and become generalized and the arthritis can be disabling. Criteria for the diagnosis of FCAS have been proposed[9] (Table 10.4). Attacks are lifelong and amyloidosis may develop. Anakinra has been shown to be effective.[10]

10.8 MUCKLE–WELL SYNDROME (MWS)

MWS is characterized by autosomal dominant transmission, very early age of onset, very frequent (several per week), short-lived

TABLE 10.4. Familial Cold Autoinflammatory Syndrome: Proposed Diagnostic Criteria[9]

Recurrent, intermittent episodes of fever and rash that primarily follow natural, experimental, or both types of generalized cold exposure
Autosomal dominant pattern of disease inheritance
Onset at <6 months of age
Duration of most attacks <24 hours
Presence of conjunctivitis associated with attacks
Absence of deafness, periorbital edema, lymphadenopathy, and serositis

TABLE 10.5. CINCA: Proposed Diagnostic Criteria[12]

A diagnosis of CINCA Syndrome can be made in a patient with a persisting urticarial rash that is migrating, of variable intensity, and often present at birth, plus at least 1 of the following:
  Symmetric arthropathy with epiphyseal and/or metaphyseal changes (early ossification of patella, with irregular ossification pattern and/or growth plate irregularities and/or irregular epiphyseal overgrowth)
  Chronic meningitis with neutrophils in the cerebrospinal fluid

Other causes of chronic, aseptic meningitis are excluded with appropriate diagnostic studies.

attacks lasting one to three days. While it has many similarities to FCAS, attacks generally occur spontaneously. Complications include amyloidosis and sensorineural deafness. Remarkable improvement has been noted in three patients from one family treated with anakinra.[11]

10.9 CHRONIC INFANTILE NEUROLOGICAL CUTANEOUS AND ARTICLUAR (CINCA) SYNDROME

The CINCA syndrome, also know as neonatal onset multisystem inflammatory disease (NOMID), is another autoinflammatory syndrome with a very early age of onset. The proposed diagnostic criteria are listed in Table 10.5.[12] The rash is often present at birth and always develops in the first few months of life. It is non-pruritic, urticarial (Figure 10.4), or papular and varies in intensity with overall disease activity. Arthropathy is marked by distinctive radiographic epiphyseal and/or metaphyseal abnormalities with premature and irregular ossification and over-

FIGURE 10.4. The CINCA picture shows the typical bossed skull and the fixed urticarial rash on the face.

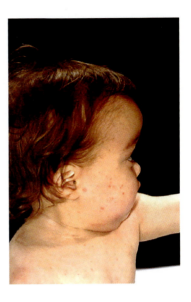

growth in about half. These radiographic changes are dramatic and characteristic and primarily affect the knees, ankles, wrists and elbows. Chronic meningitis, with neutrophilic pleocytosis, is present in most children. Chronic headache, vomiting from raised intracranial pressure, delayed closure of the anterior fontanelle frontal bossing and multiple sensory abnormalities are common. Cerebral atrophy and cerebral calcifications seen on brain imaging may occur. Ocular abnormalities include both anterior and posterior uveitis, papilledema and, rarely, blindness. Sensorineural deafness and hoarse voice are frequent. Developmental delay and growth delay are both common. There have been reports of dramatic response to anakinra.[11]

10.10 KEY POINTS
- Autoinflammatory syndromes should be suspected in young children with recurrent fevers seemingly unresponsive to antibiotics.
- Family history is extremely helpful in making the diagnosis, but the disease may also be sporadic as the result of a spontaneous mutation.
- Consider autoinflammatory syndromes in the Differential Diagnosis of recurrent fevers when infections, malignancies and inflammatory "connective tissue diseases" have been excluded.

- Genetic testing is available for the majority of the known Periodic Fever Syndromes.
- Early treatment may prevent long-term morbidity.

References

1. Frenkel J, Kuis W. Overt and occult rheumatic diseases: the child with chronic fever. *Best Pract Res Clin Rheumatol.* 2002;16:443–469.

2. Ancient missense mutations in a new member of the RoRet gene family are likely to cause familial Mediterranean fever. The International FMF Consortium. *Cell.* 1997;90:797–807.

3. Zemer D, Livneh A, Danon YL et al. Long-term colchicine treatment in children with familial Mediterranean fever. *Arthritis Rheum.* 1991;34:973–977.

4. Padeh S, Brezniak N, Zemer D et al. Periodic fever, aphthous stomatitis, pharyngitis, and adenopathy syndrome: clinical characteristics and outcome. *J Pediatr.* 1999;135:98–101.

5. Drenth JP, Haagsma CJ, van der Meer JW. Hyperimmunoglobuline-mia D and periodic fever syndrome. The clinical spectrum in a series of 50 patients. International Hyper-IgD Study Group. *Medicine (Baltimore).* 1994;73:133–144.

6. Takada K, Aksentijevich I, Mahadevan V et al. Favorable preliminary experience with etanercept in two patients with the hyperimmunoglobulinemia D and periodic fever syndrome. *Arthritis Rheum.* 2003;48:2645–2651.

7. Hull KM, Drewe E, Aksentijevich I et al. The TNF receptor-associated periodic syndrome (TRAPS): emerging concepts of an autoinflammatory disorder. *Medicine (Baltimore).* 2002;81:349–368.

8. Aksentijevich I, Nowak M, Mallah M et al. De novo CIAS1 mutations, cytokine activation, and evidence for genetic heterogeneity in patients with neonatal-onset multisystem inflammatory disease (NOMID): a new member of the expanding family of pyrin-associated autoinflammatory diseases. *Arthritis Rheum.* 2002;46:3340–3348.

9. Hoffman HM, Wanderer AA, Broide DH. Familial cold autoinflammatory syndrome: Phenotype and genotype of an autosomal dominant periodic fever. *J Allergy Clin Immunol.* 2001;108:615–620.

10. Hoffman HM, Rosengren S, Boyle DL et al. Prevention of cold-associated acute inflammation in familial cold autoinflammatory syndrome by interleukin-1 receptor antagonist. *Lancet.* 2004;364:1779–1785.

11. Goldbach-Mansky R, Dailey NJ, Canna SW et al. Neonatal-onset multisystem inflammatory disease responsive to IL-6beta inhibition. *New Eng J Med.* 2006;355:581–592.

12. Prieur AM. A recently recognised chronic inflammatory disease of early onset characterised by the triad of rash, central nervous system involvement and arthropathy. *Clin Exp Rheumatol.* 2001;19:103–106.

Chapter 11
Acute Rheumatic Fever and Post Streptococcal Arthritis

11.1 INTRODUCTION
Acute rheumatic fever (ARF) has been known for centuries and is one of the unique rheumatic diseases that is causally related to prior pharyngitis due to Group A β hemolytic Streptococci. Post streptococcal arthritis (PSRA) has more recently been defined. Neither follows streptococcal infection of the skin, which can cause an immune complex mediated glomerulonephritis.

11.2 ACUTE RHEUMATIC FEVER

11.2.1 Definition
In 1944, Jones established criteria for diagnosing ARF that has undergone several revisions. The 1992 criteria are shown on Table 11.1.[1]

11.2.2 Epidemiology
The incidence in developed countries is as low as <1 per 100,000 and in undeveloped countries (and certain at risk populations) over 100 per 100,000. It is more common in Pacific islanders, Australian aborigines, in South America, the Indian subcontinent and the Middle East. Localized outbreaks are not unusual in developed countries. It most typically affects children aged 5 to 15 years old, and is rare under the age of 4 years.[2,3]

11.2.3 Etiology
The inciting agent is Group A β hemolytic Streptococci pharyngitis in a susceptible host. Streptococci M protein and hyaluronate cross react with human myocardium, myosin, brain, cartilage, and synovial fluid.[4] There are about 100 M serotypes, only a handful are rheumatogenic. The host factors may include having HLA DRB1*16 and a β-lymphocyte cell surface marker known as D8/17. The latter has been reported in up to 99% of children with ARF and only 14% of normals.[5]

TABLE 11.1. Jones Criteria to Establish the Diagnosis of Acute Rheumatic Fever (ARF): Requires 2 of the Major Criteria or 1 Major and 2 Minor Criteria

Major (% typically affected)	Minor
Carditis (50%)	Prolonged PR interval
Arthritis (migratory) (70%)	Arthralgia (cannot use if also
Erythema marginatum (<5%)	has arthritis)
Nodules (subcutaneous) (<5%)	Increased ESR or CRP
Chorea (15%)	Fever

11.2.4 Clinical Manifestations

Arthritis affects about 70% of children with ARF (Table 11.1). The arthritis is typically migratory, lasting hours to a few days in any given joint, with large joints preferentially involved. It is associated with extreme pain and even redness that responses rapidly to aspirin or other nonsteroidal anti-inflammatory drugs (NSAIDs). Large joints are more commonly involved. The carditis typically causes an endocarditis with involvement of the mitral value (and not infrequently the aortic, but only rarely the tricuspid and pulmonary). Myocarditis with failure and pericarditis can occur early on and is manifest in about 5% of children with ARF. Erythema marginatum is manifest early on as a serpiginous, nonpruritic erythematous rash, usually centrally located and migratory. Early in the course of ARF the minor manifestations are present, including fever, generally over 39°C (102°F) and arthralgia. Although not part of the criterion, abdominal pain responsive to NSAIDs and epistaxis can occur. Generally, two to three weeks later, painless subcutaneous nodules on the extensors surfaces (hands, feet, back and occiput) may develop and last about three weeks; they are associated with severe carditis. The last manifestation to arise, two to six months later, is chorea (St. Vitus' dance) and may be the only evidence of ARF. It is much more common in girls, and is manifest by choreiform movements of the arms, face and tongue. A rhythmic hand squeezing (milk maid grip) is typical as is emotional lability and obsessive-compulsive behaviors. Chorea is worse with anxiety and resolves during sleep. The movements last six weeks to six months.[6]

11.2.5 Laboratory Features

It is imperative to establish a prior streptococcal infection. The antistreptolysin O (ASO) titre is elevated in only 80% of children with ARF. Adding a second test, generally the anti-deoxyribonuclease B (anti-DNase B) will capture over 95% of children with prior streptococcal infections. The streptozyme test is not sensitive or specific enough to be routinely used to establish, by itself, either ARF or PSRA. Other streptococcal antigens are not routinely tested for in most hospitals (anti-nicotinamide adenine dinucleotidase (NADase) and antihyaluronidase). Antibodies should rise at least four-fold between acute and convalescent sera, but the criteria state only a two-fold increase or fall is sufficient if the initial values are not convincing of a prior streptococcal infection.

11.2.6 Establishing the Diagnosis
The diagnosis requires evidence of prior streptococcal disease and two major or one major and two minor criteria. Exceptions are chorea, the presence of rheumatic heart disease, and an illness like ARF in someone who has already suffered rheumatic heart damage so the presence of active carditis is not certain.[1]

11.2.7 Treatment
Children with ARF should be treated initially for streptococcus and then prophylactic antibiotic should be given according to Table 11.2. Some studies suggest high-risk patients should have parental prophylaxis every three weeks rather than every four weeks.[7]

11.2.8 Outcome
The major morbidity and mortality from ARF arises from heart damage, although up to 80% with long-term prophylaxis will resolve the valvular lesion.[8] Recurrent ARF is characterized with an increased incidence of severe carditis.

TABLE 11.2. Prophylactic Treatment to Prevent Recurrent Streptococcal Infection

Preferred	
Penicillin G Benzathine	1.2 Million Units IM q 3–4 weeks
	600,000 Units IM q 3–4 weeks if ≤27 kg
Alternative	
Penicillin V	250 mg PO BID
Sulfadiazine	500 mg PO q day if ≤27 kg
	1 gram PO q day if >27 kg
If allergic to Penicillin and Sulfadiazine	
Erythromycin	250 mg PO BID

11.3 POST STREPTOCOCCAL REACTIVE ARTHRITIS (PSRA)

Post streptococcal arthritis is a reactive arthritis that differs from the arthritis of ARF. It is nonmigratory, lasts longer, does not respond as well to aspirin, and typically involves both small and large joints.[9–11] These children do not have carditis or other major manifestations.

11.3.1 Epidemiology

There are no good epidemiologic studies of PSRA, but in North America it is more common than ARF. It generally affects children late in childhood, adolescence, and into adulthood, without a sex or ethnic predilection. It follows group A, C, and G streptococcal pharyngitis. It may be more common in children with HLA DRB1*01.

11.3.2 Clinical Manifestations

Most children with PSRA have polyarthritis, although oligoarthritis and monarthritis may occur. Axial disease may occur, more typically in those who are HLA-B27 positive.

11.3.3 Establishing the Diagnosis

The diagnosis requires evidence of prior streptococcal disease, the lack of major criteria for ARF, and nonmigratory, nonfleeting arthritis.

11.3.4 Laboratory Features

Attempt to establish prior streptococcal disease as for ARF above should be made. Additionally, we advocate searching for major and minor manifestations of ARF, especially obtaining an electrocardiogram and echocardiogram.

11.3.5 Treatment

Children with PSRA should be treated initially for streptococcus. Prophylaxis is controversial even though approximately 5% of children will have silent carditis and, over time, a mitral regurgitation murmur will be appreciated. Some physicians will give prophylactic antibiotics for 1 to 2 years and then, if an echocardiogram is normal, stop and watch carefully.[11]

The arthritis is more chronic than ARF and not as responsive to NSAIDs, although they do give symptomatic relief. Intraarticular corticosteroids in those with a few joints involved will quickly resolve the arthritis in most. Some children will require a disease modifying agent, as in JIA (see Chapter 3). Physical therapy is beneficial in children with joint and muscle tightness.

11.3.6 Outcome

The arthritis of PSRA is longer lasting than ARF, but in most cases will resolve in 2 to 8 months. Rarely children can have protracted arthritis.

References

1. Guidelines for the diagnosis of rheumatic fever. Jones Criteria, 1992 update. Special Writing Group of the Committee on Rheumatic Fever, Endocarditis, and Kawasaki Disease of the Council on Cardiovascular Disease in the Young of the American Heart Association. [Erratum in JAMA 1993 Jan 27;269:476]. *JAMA*. 1992;268:2069–2073.
2. Amigo MC, Martinez-Lavin M, Reyes PA. Acute rheumatic fever. *Rheum Dis Clin North Am*. 1993;19:333–350.
3. Tani LY, Veasey LG, Minigill et al. Rheumatic fever in children younger than 5 years: is the presentation different? *Pediatrics*. 2003;112:1065–1068.
4. Bisno AL, Brito MO, Collins CM. Molecular basis of group A streptococcal virulence. *Lancet Infect Dis*. 2003;3:191–200.
5. Harel L, Zehana A, Kodman Y et al. Presence of the d8/17 B-cell marker in children with rheumatic fever in Israel. *Clin Genet*. 2002;61:293–298.
6. Bonthius DJ, Karacay B. Sydenham's chorea: not gone and not forgotten. *Semin Pediatr Neurol*. 2003;10:11–19.
7. Thatai D, Turi ZG. Current guidelines for the treatment of patients with rheumatic fever. *Drugs*. 1999;57:545–555.
8. Feldman T. Rheumatic heart disease. *Curr Opin Cardiol*. 1996;11:126–130.
9. Ayoub EM, Majeed HA. Poststreptococcal reactive arthritis. *Curr Opin Rheumatol*. 2000;12:306–310.
10. Ahmed S, Ayoub EM. Poststreptococcal reactive arthritis. *Pediat Infect Dis J*. 2001;20:1081–1082.
11. Shulman ST, Ayoub EM. Poststreptococcal reactive arthritis. *Curr Opin Rheumatol*. 2002;14:562–565.

Part III

Noninflammatory Rheumatologic Diseases

Chapter 12
Noninflammatory Mechanical Pain Syndromes

12.1 INTRODUCTION
Musculoskeletal pain is the presenting complaint in 20% of physician visits. Most are short-lived and resolve uneventfully. We will discuss three major categories in this section, because they may mimic rheumatic conditions, or may come to the rheumatologist due to the perplexing nature of the condition for diagnosis and treatment, or are associated with significant morbidity. These include mechanical conditions (mostly orthopedic), the amplified musculoskeletal pain syndromes (see Chapter 13), and hereditary syndromes affecting the musculoskeletal system (see Chapter 14).

12.2 BENIGN HYPERMOBILITY SYNDROME (BHMS)
Up to 20% of girls are hypermobile, as are 10% of boys. Adult patients with hypermobility, as defined by Beighton, usually have 6 out of 9 possible abnormalities on examination and this has been validated for Dutch children (Table 12.1).[1] (Figures 12.1 to 12.8). Children with pain due to benign hypermobility syndrome usually complain of pain in the evening, or at night after going to bed. The pain can awaken the child and can be severe enough to cause crying and screaming. It is usually located in the legs, frequently behind the knee and is helped by massage, analgesics, and warmth. It is relatively short lived and most notable, the child is without stiffness or complaint in the morning and there is no gelling (stiffness after rest, such as a nap or long car ride).[2] The symptomatic child with BHMS often has poor neuromuscular control. Asymmetric hypermobility in the weight bearing joints (e.g., hypermobile knees and not hips or ankles) can also lead to similar symptoms.

The examination is notable only for hypermobility, and joint swelling is not present. The typical age for BHMS is 3 to 8, it is rare in adolescents and most children thought to have growing pain in the older age range usually have enthesitis (see

TABLE 12.1. Beighton Scale for Hypermobility

	Score
Able to touch thumb to forearm, right and left	2
Hyperextend fifth MCP so finger parallels forearm, right and left	2
Greater than 10° hyperextension of elbows, right and left	2
Greater than 10° hyperextension of knees, right and left	2
Able to touch palms to floor with knees straight	1

*A score of six or more findings define hypermobility.[1]

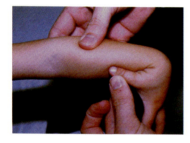

FIGURE 12.1. Demonstration of hypermobile thumb.

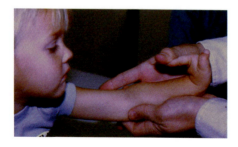

FIGURE 12.2. Demonstration of hypermobile MCPs.

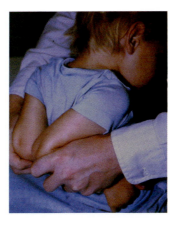

FIGURE 12.3. Demonstration of hypermobile shoulders.

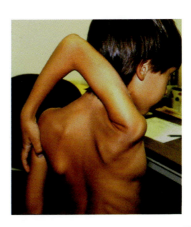

FIGURE 12.4. Demonstration of extremely hypermobile shoulders.

12

Chapter 3). Features of Marfan syndrome and Ehlers–Danlos should be sought in any patient with hypermobility, since further consultation would be indicated. Some classify typical benign hypermobility syndrome, as described above, as Ehlers–Danlos type III. However, the more serious forms of Ehlers–Danlos syndrome are characterised by extreme hypermobility, loose skin (check over the forehead and sternum as well as the elbows and

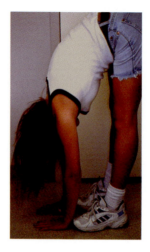

FIGURE 12.5. Demonstration of hypermobile hips.

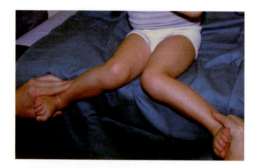

FIGURE 12.6. Demonstration of hypermobile hips.

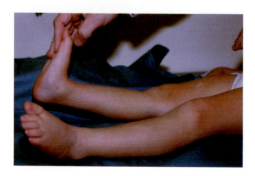

FIGURE 12.7. Demonstration of hypermobile knees.

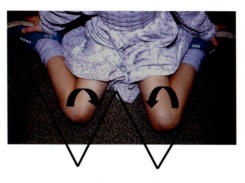

FIGURE 12.8. Demonstration of hypermobile hips and knees sitting in W.

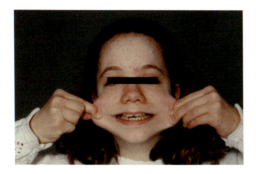

FIGURE 12.9. Exceptionally elastic skin of a girl with Erhlers–Danlos syndrome.

knees) (Figure 12.9) and thin, cigarette paper scars.[3] Marfan syndrome is notable for arachnodactyly, high arched palate, long arms (the arm span times 1.03 is greater than the height), disproportional long lower body segment, pectus carinatum or excavatum, and sparse subcutaneous body fat.[4] Children with Ehlers-Danlos or Marfan syndrome should have a genetic consultation and many require surveillance for aortic aneurysms, and cardiac or ophthalmologic complications.

The treatment of hypermobility is reassurance and, if pain is frequent, an evening dose of either acetaminophen or ibuprofen can dramatically improve the evening life of the family. Parents should be warned to acknowledge the pain and give some measure of comfort (massage, reassurance to the child), but not unnecessary secondary gain (stories, sleeping with the parents, facilitating bedtime avoidance). Progressive exercises to improve balance and muscle control of the hypermobile joints are beneficial, as are orthotics in children with severe pes planus.

Some children with typical hypermobility pain are not hypermobile. These children have often been labelled as having growing pains, although this term is a misnomer as it has nothing to do with the rate of growth and we prefer the term benign nocturnal musculoskeletal pains of childhood. It is worth checking whether the symptomatic joint is next to a hypermobile joint, as this could often put undue stress on the nonhypermobile joint. The treatment is the same as for hypermobility, but we would recommend rechecking the joint examination in 3 to 5 months to make sure subclinical illness has not evolved into arthritis or enthesitis.

12.3 OSGOOD–SCHLATTER SYNDROME

Osgood–Schlatter syndrome is due to microavulsion fractures of the tibial tubercle. The infrapatellar tendon pulls on the relative weak tibial tubercle entheses leading to microavulsion. The bone remodels as the tendon continues to pull so a noticeable bump forms at the tibial tubercle. It occurs in the rapidly growing adolescent, usually 8 to 13 years old. Boys outnumber girls 3:1. Patients with Osgood-Schlatter syndrome are very tender over the tibial tubercle (more tender than enthesitis) and frequently are unable to kneel. It is bilateral in 30% (Figure 12.10). Treat-

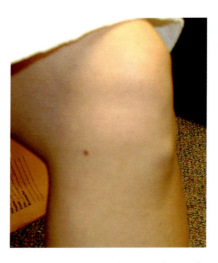

FIGURE 12.10. In Osgood–Schlatter disease, the tendon is thickened, often associated with a bursa and a very tender and enlarged tibial tubercle.

ment is rest and symptomatic care. The diagnosis is made clinically, but if severe and unremitting, a radiograph can ascertain if a pseudoarthrosis has formed, which will need surgical attention.[5]

12.4 SINDING–LARSEN–JOHANNSON SYNDROME

An analogous situation to Osgood–Schlatter syndrome can occur at the inferior pole of the patella, called Sinding–Larsen–Johannson syndrome. It, too, is more frequent in early adolescent boys, especially athletes. It is more painful than enthesitis (see Chapter 3). It is exacerbated by running, stairs and kneeling, and there is usually swelling. The treatment is rest and symptomatic care. In severe cases, a cast or splint can help enforce rest and hasten healing.

12.5 SEVER SYNDROME

Sever syndrome is an apophysitis of the calcaneous, usually in children aged 8 to 13 years. It is more common in boys, 2 : 1, and causes activity related heel pain. It is characterized by point tenderness at the corner of the calcaneous. Heel cups help most of the time and, if needed, acetaminophen or ibuprofen may be administered.

12.6 OSTEONECROSIS

Children are susceptible to idiopathic osteonecrosis in a variety of bones. These may be due to trauma to the growing bone. Eponyms are frequently used, depending on the location. The more common areas of osteonecrosis involve the lunate (Kienböck), second metatarsal head (Freiberg), proximal tibia (Blount), tarsal navicular (Köhler), and vertebral epiphysis (Scheuermann). Treatment is usually supportive and may require temporary splinting and avoiding activities that lead to trauma to the area involved (such as karate with Kienböck).

12.7 COSTOCHRONDRITIS

One of the most common causes of chest pain in older adolescents is costochrondritis, inflammation of the cartilaginous junction of the rib and sternum. It is more common in girls. It is termed Tietze syndrome if swelling is present. It is usually post viral and can last for months. It is aggravated with trauma and even from lying prone on a hard surface, such as the floor, while reading.

12

12.8 EPICONDYLITIS

Point tenderness of the medial epicondyle (golfer's or little league elbow) or lateral epicondyle (tennis elbow) is an overuse injury seen in adolescent athletes. It causes local aches and is characterised by point tenderness that increases with resisted motion. Conservative measures, such as ice, counterforce bracing, and rest usually suffice, although some patients need NSAIDs or local corticosteroid injection.

12.9 HIP PAIN

Isolated hip pain is of special urgency due to the inability to feel joint swelling, the susceptibility of the hip to various conditions and infection, and the importance of hip in function. Differential diagnoses include the following:

12.9.1 Septic Hip

Septic arthritis of the hip is not uncommon and requires intravenous antibiotics and drainage. It is most common below the age of five; boys outnumber girls 2:1. Staphylococcus aureus is the most common infectious organism. It causes acute pain that is extreme and usually causes immobility of the hip and prevents weight bearing. It is accompanied by fever, malaise, and elevated acute phase reactants. It is usually not confused with the rheumatic or mechanical conditions, although an occasional child with oligoarthritis of the hip or toxic synovitis will need to be investigated for potential septic hip.

12.9.2 Toxic Synovitis (Transient Synovitis, Observation Hip)

Toxic synovitis affecting the hip is more common in boys aged 3 to 10 years, and frequently follows an upper respiratory tract infection. It is neither as tender, nor as limiting of mobility, as a septic joint, and the acute phase reactants are normal or only mildly elevated. If infection is suspected, joint aspiration is indicated. Normally it can be treated with NSAIDs and rest over time. Most symptoms resolve within a week. Frequent recurrence should alert the physician to evolving enthesitis arthritis.

12.10 LEGG–CALVÉ–PERTHES

Legg–Calvé–Perthes is an avascular necrosis of the femoral head usually seen in children aged 4 to 10 years. It is more frequent in boys, 4:1, and is bilateral in 20%. The complaint is frequently limp and not painful. It is diagnosed by plain radiography, and there are five radiologic stages: (1) cessation of capital femora epiphyseal growth, (2) subchondral fracture, (3) resorption (frag-

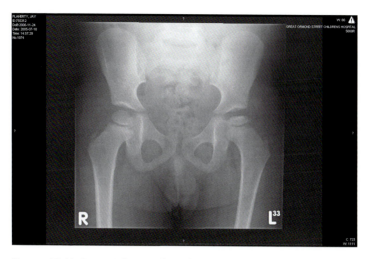

FIGURE 12.11. Legg–Calvé–Perthes of the left hip.

mentation), (4) reossification, and (5) healed or residual stage (Figure 12.11). It is a self-limited condition and the goal of treatment is to contain the femoral head within the acetabulum so that the latter acts as a mould, preventing further long-term damage. Orthopedic expertise should be obtained. Prognosis is based primarily on the age of onset, with younger children doing much better, and secondarily the degree of femoral head collapse.[6]

12.11 SLIPPED CAPITAL FEMORAL EPIPHYSIS

Slipped capital femora epiphysis (SCFE) is a fracture through the femoral head epiphysis. SCFE occurs most frequently in obese adolescents, but can also afflict those who have delayed skeletal maturation, or who are tall and thin with a recent growth spurt. It may have an underlying endocrinologic cause, especially hypothyroidism. It can have an acute or chronic onset, so it may not present as an acutely painful hip. A new limp with limited rotation of the hip should prompt radiographs, anterior-posterior and frog leg lateral projections. Widening of the physis without slippage is the earliest sign of SCFE, but as the slip progresses, the head remains in the acetabulum and the femoral neck rotates anteriorly. Urgent orthopedic consultation is indicated.

12.12 IDIOPATHIC CHONDROLYSIS OF THE HIP

Idiopathic chondrolysis is characterised by progressive loss of cartilage in adolescents, affects more girls than boys and has a slight predilection in Africans and African Americans. The diagnosis is made radiographically, with the exclusion of other conditions, usually requiring biopsy. Treatment is symptomatic and ultimately surgical.

12.13 LABORATORY TESTS

In children presenting with most of the above conditions, no laboratory tests are indicated. If there is concern about an early infection then acute phase reactants can be checked (CBC, ESR, or CRP). Rheumatologic disease laboratory studies should not be done. Fifteen percent of normal children will have a nonspecific positive ANA test that will lead to unnecessary referral, expense, and worry.[7]

Imaging studies are universally required for hip symptoms since SCFE needs immediate attention and Legg–Calvé–Perthes need not be treated as arthritis of the hip. Other radiographs are indicated if an osteonecrosis or traumatic injury is suspected. Radiographs do not help with the early identification of arthritis although many rheumatologists like to establish a baseline to compare to subsequent studies to determine the rate of joint damage. Ultrasound, scintigraphy and magnet resonance studies have their place and are discussed when indicated throughout this text.

References

1. Beighton P, Solomon L, Soskolne CL. Articular mobility in an African population, *Ann Rheum Dis*. 1973;32:413–418.
2. El-Garf AK, Mahmoud GA, Mahgoub EH. Hypermobility among Egyptian children: prevalence and features. *J Rheumatol*. 1998;25:1003–1005.
3. Byers PH. Ehlers-Danlos syndrome: recent advances and current understanding of the clinical and genetic heterogeneity. *J Invest Dermatol*. 1994;103:47S–52S.
4. De Paepe A, Devereux RB, Dietz HC et al. Revised diagnostic criteria for the Marfan syndrome. *Am J Med Genet*. 1996;62:417–426.
5. Orava S, Malinen L, Karpakka J et al. Results of surgical treatment of unresolved Osgood-Schlatter lesion. *Ann Chir Gynaecol*. 2000;89(suppl):298–302.
6. Wall EJ. Legg–Calvé–Perthes' disease. *Curr Opin Pediatr*. 1999;11:76–79.
7. Allen RC, Dewez P, Stuart L et al. Antinuclear antibodies using HEp-2 cells in normal children and in children with common infections. *J Paediatr Child Health*. 1991;27:39–42.

Chapter 13
Amplified Musculoskeletal Pain

13.1 INTRODUCTION

An increasing number of children have various forms of amplified musculoskeletal pain. These children are more disabled than children with arthritis and they and their families suffer intensely. In addition to their pain, frequently they are isolated from peers and are commonly told by medical professionals that they are faking it or that it does not hurt all that much. These children are very challenging but quite rewarding.

DEFINITION. *Chronic musculoskeletal pain increased out of proportion to the known stimulus.*

13.1.1 The Name

There are multiple manifestations of amplified musculoskeletal pain, usually defined by the location or presence of autonomic dysfunction. Two broad categories are children with localised pain and those with diffuse pain.[1] Of those with localised pain, the most easily recognised is complex regional pain syndrome type 1 (CRPS1), formerly known as reflex sympathetic dystrophy.[2] These children have overt autonomic dysfunction manifest by coolness or cyanosis of the limb and occasionally increased perspiration or edema. Many children have very localized pain amplification but do not have autonomic signs. Of the children with diffuse pain, the most written about is fibromyalgia (although many physicians do not use this term for children since it may differ from adult fibromyalgia). There are two different criteria for fibromyalgia. The American College of Rheumatology criteria requires 11 of 18 trigger points on the body to be painful (Figure 13.1) along with 3 months of widespread pain.[3] The criteria of Yunus and Masi require either 4 or 5 painful trigger points and multiple related symptoms (Table 13.1).[4] Determining whether a trigger point is painful or not is highly subjective and varies between examiners and over time.

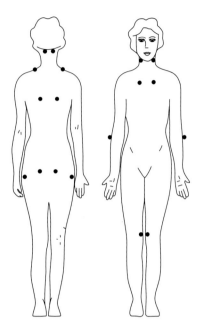

FIGURE 13.1. The trigger points of fibromyalgia.

TABLE 13.1. The Yunus and Masi Criteria for Fibromyalgia* in Children[4]

Major
  Generalized musculoskeletal aching at 3 or more sites for 3 or
    more months
  Absence of underlying condition or cause
  Normal laboratory tests
  Five or more typical tender points

Minor
  Chronic anxiety or tension
  Fatigue
  Poor sleep
  Chronic headaches
  Irritable bowel syndrome
  Subjective soft tissue swelling
  Numbness
  Pain modulation by physical activities
  Pain modulation by weather factors
  Pain modulation by anxiety/stress

*Fibromyalgia defined as present if the subject has all 4 major criteria
and 3 minor criteria, or first 3 major criteria, 4 tender points, and 5 minor
criteria.

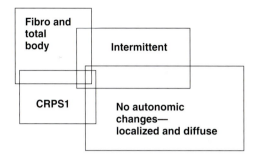

FIGURE 13.2. The overlapping nature of the various forms of amplified musculoskeletal pain in children.

Not all children with diffuse pain have painful trigger points and so do not satisfy the criteria for fibromyalgia. Additionally, there are children with intermittent localized or diffuse pains or overlapping features of the above, e.g., a cool blue foot and total body pain. Figure 13.2 displays the overlapping nature of these conditions.

13.1.2 Epidemiology

There are no specific studies of the incidence of amplified musculoskeletal pain in children. Studies of normal schoolchildren have found 1.2% to 6% fulfil criteria for fibromyalgia and 7.5% report widespread musculoskeletal pain. Children with amplified musculoskeletal pain make up approximately 10% of children in pediatric rheumatic disease clinics and it is the impression of many that the incidence is increasing.[5–7]

The average age of onset is preteen to early teen. It is rare below the age of seven years so diagnosing amplified musculoskeletal pain in young children needs to be done with much circumspection. However, children as young as two and three years old have developed it.

Girls are overrepresented at a ratio of at least 5:1. This may be because girls have lower pain thresholds and report pain more frequently than boys, however, boys and girls with chronic pain do not differ in physician utilization.

Most children with amplified musculoskeletal pain are Caucasian and there is a suspicion that the majority is from the upper socioeconomic levels, however no race or economic level is spared.

13

13.1.3 Etiology

The etiology is unknown but it seems related to trauma, illness, or psychological distress. Most pediatric rheumatologists think the psychological distress plays a significant role in most but not all cases. Whether cause or effect, most children have such pain and dysfunction that this, itself, inflicts psychological havoc on the child and family. Genetic factors have been implicated in fibromyalgia and CRPS1 and a very weak association has been made between fibromyalgia and hypermobility (see Chapter 12). It is likely that there is a combination of both intrinsic factors, such as individual pain threshold, female sex, and coping strategies and extrinsic factors, such as previous pain experiences, social stresses, modeling of chronic pain behaviors, and central and peripheral pain mechanisms that work in concert to give rise to amplified musculoskeletal pain.[8]

13.2 CLINICAL MANIFESTATIONS

Although each child is different, there are unifying threads in the history and physical examination to establish the pattern for most. The archetypal patient is a mature and accomplished adolescent girl who suffers a minor injury or illness and then has increasing pain and dysfunction over several days to months. The pain may be localised, with or without signs of autonomic dysfunction, or diffuse. Sometimes it begins as localised pain and spreads. Allodynia is common and clothing bumps while riding in the car, and even the wind hitting their skin causes pain. Some children, usually those with diffuse pain, will have multiple somatic complaints, which help define fibromyalgia by the Yunus and Masi criteria (Table 13.1). The child will report very high levels of pain (10 out of 10) usually with an incongruent, cheerful affect and severe dysfunction. They will be severely incapacitated. Multiple physician visits and therapeutic failures are common.

Autonomic signs seen in CRPS1 usually consist of coolness and cyanosis (Figure 13.3). These signs may not be manifest at rest but become apparent after exercising the limb. Occasionally there is increased perspiration or dystrophic skin (Figure 13.4).

Allodynia is tested by either light touch or gentle pinching of a fold of skin. The area of allodynia may vary in location on repeated testing.

Painful trigger points can be found in those with fibromyalgia. These points are reported as painful, not tender or sore, with 3 to 4 kgs of digital pressure. The points are shown in Figure 13.1. Control points should also be tested such as the forehead, thumbnail, shaft of the tibia, and outer third of the clavicle.[9] Those with

FIGURE 13.3. Cyanosis and slight swelling in an adolescent girl with CRPS1 of the left foot: It was extremely tender to light touch.

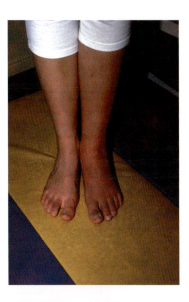

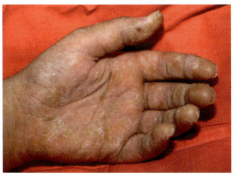

FIGURE 13.4. Dystrophic skin changes in an adolescent with CRPS1.

painful control points are, perhaps, better defined as having total body pain.

Conversion symptoms are not infrequent; numbness is the most common, followed by a bizarre gait, paralysis, or abnormal shaking or tremors. Dizziness is not uncommon, but vestibular function tests are normal.[10]

13.2.1 Laboratory Tests

All laboratory blood and urine tests are normal. Radiographs may show osteoporosis and bone scintigraphy is usually normal

13

but it can show decreased uptake, especially in CRPS1 (or spotty increased uptake characteristic of adult CRPS1).[11] Magnetic resonance images can show edema, but the anatomy is otherwise intact.

13.2.2 Diagnostic Pitfalls

The most common diagnosis made in children thought to have an amplified musculoskeletal pain is spondyloarthropathy, since one doesn't generally check for enthesitis (Chapter 3). Malignancies, usually spinal cord tumors, are the most serious condition missed, so a detailed neurological examination is mandatory. Arthritis has been mistaken for amplified musculoskeletal pain, but it is usually obvious on examination. Some children with arthritis will have, in addition, an amplified musculoskeletal pain syndrome so both ailments need to be independently addressed. Rarely, undetected thyroid disease will be manifest as diffuse pain.

13.2.3 Disease Activity

Initially and during follow-up, there needs to be ongoing assessment of pain and dysfunction. Self-report, such as 0 to 10 on a verbal scale or marking a visual analogue scale, is adequate to measure pain. Functional measures usually consist of a questionnaire inquiring about a standard set of age-appropriate activities, but, in practice, asking about school attendance, waking endurance, chores and participation in recreational activities will suffice.

13.3 TREATMENT

It is paramount to establish a trusting relationship with the child and family. Foremost, believe that the child is in pain since these children have been given both verbal and nonverbal messages that the pain is all in their head or that they are malingering. It is useful to explain the pain in terms of sympathetically mediated pain amplification (Figure 13.5); this reinforces the reality of the pain, gives an understandable reason for the pain, and is a mechanism in which to introduce the treatment strategy.[12]

Discontinue all medical investigations. Too many families are convinced that some diagnosis has been overlooked and that a test (even if done previously and was normal) will establish a diagnosis.

All medications need to be discontinued. Some children who are on antidepressants for depression or anxiety disorders will need to continue, but those treated with antidepressants for pain

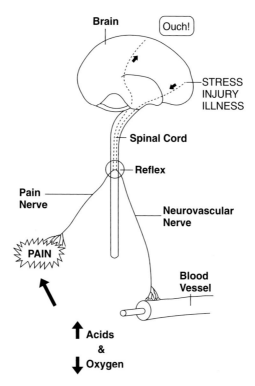

FIGURE 13.5. Working model to explain amplified musuloskeletal pain via sympathetically mediated tissue ischemia.

should stop taking the drug. Some medications need to be tapered, specifically, opioids should be tapered about 10% a day and gabapentin over 2 to 3 weeks, depending on the dose. Tramadol binds to μ opioid receptors so, if on a high dose, it should also be tapered.

There are no controlled studies of the vast number of reported treatments for the various forms of amplified musculoskeletal pain. Treatments have ranged from pain medications, antidepressants, gabapentin, transcutaneous nerve stimulation, nerve blocks and sympathectomy (for CRPS1), epidural catheters for continuous infusion including pain pumps, lidocaine and opioid patches, acupuncture, cognitive-behavior therapy, psychotherapy, and exercise therapy.

Most agree that exercise therapy is helpful and it is associated with the best long-term outcomes in all forms of amplified musculoskeletal pain and we have found it the most helpful with the longest lasting results.[13,14] The nature of the exercise therapy is different to that which most physical and occupational therapists are accustomed to. The primary goal is to restore function so the program is very intense and directed at doing normal and aerobic activities, such as jumping, stairs, walking speed and endurance, sports drills, and carrying loads. Pain is not directly treated and is ignored as much as possible during the exercising. The vast majority will resolve all pain once full function has been restored. Allodynia is treated with desensitization with towel and lotion rubs. Many children will require up to 5 hours of exercise therapy daily, on average, for 2 to 3 weeks. Additionally, most children will show improvement in their mood, sleep, energy level, and other somatic complaints.

In addition to exercise, the psychodynamics of the child and family should be evaluated, since most families and children, but not all, will have significant psychological problems that can be helped with individual, family, or marital therapy.[15,16]

Sleep deserves special mention, but addressing sleep problems does not resolve the somatic symptoms. Many children with amplified musculoskeletal pain have a sleep complaint (not a true sleep disorder) and good sleep hygiene is helpful. This includes going to bed only when one is sleepy, not engaging in other activities in bed such as reading or watching television, eliminating caffeine, relaxation techniques, elimination of napping and having a routine for sleeping and waking.

Traditional (nonallopathic) treatments are frequently sought, but there is no data regarding benefit. These include herbal therapy, massage, magnet therapy, homeopathy, reflexology, and aromatherapy to name a few, but only rarely is any sustained benefit reported. We cannot recommend any and, like allopathic medications, we discontinue them once the diagnosis is clear.

13.4 OUTCOME

The outcome may vary on the form of amplified musculoskeletal pain; however, long-term studies in children are few. Most children, 92% of 103 children, with CRPS1 treated with an intense exercise program resolved all signs and symptoms and 88% were well after 5 years.[14] Less than half of 70 children with CRPS1, treated with drugs, blocks, and moderate exercise, resolved all symptoms; no long-term outcome is reported.[17]

Children with diffuse pain or fibromyalgia may have more long-term pain, depending on the treatment and study.[16,18] However, 11 of 15 schoolchildren identified on screening to have fibromyalgia resolved their fibromyalgia after 30 months.[19] Cognitive-behavior therapy alone was used in 5 girls with fibromyalgia and 4 reported no pain 10 months later.[20]

Children with amplified musculoskeletal pain may go on to develop other targets for pain such as headaches and abdominal pain.[8] Additionally, nonpainful outcomes take on many forms of unresolved psychological issues and include conversion reactions, eating disorders, school avoidance, suicide attempts, and acting out behaviors.

13.5 SUMMARY

Children with amplified musculoskeletal pain suffer significant pain and disability and need compassionate care that should include accurate diagnosis, as well as a consistent evaluative and therapeutic approach. The psychological aspects of these conditions should be formally assessed. Intense exercise therapy, along with desensitisation, is of great benefit to most. Normal function should be restored at a minimum. School attendance should be mandatory and social activities and sports encouraged. If pain continues, then either pain coping skills using cognitive behavioral therapy, or more formal psychotherapy should be pursued. Pharmacological agents should be limited to specific indications, not pain control. Children with amplified musculoskeletal pain and their families can be challenging, but the benefit gained by all is quite rewarding.

KEY POINTS

- Have a high index of suspicion for the presence of amplified musculoskeletal pain especially in:
  - Adolescent girls
    - Mature beyond years
    - Accomplished
    - Perfectionistic
    - Pleaser
  - Prolonged school absence due to pain
  - Marked dysfunction
  - Pain is continuing to get worse
  - Normal examination except pain
    - No enthesitis or arthritis
    - Normal neurological exam

- ○ Localised pain on examination
  - Allodynia (variable border)
  - Autonomic signs
  - Incongruent affect
  - La belle indifference
- ○ Widespread pain on examination
  - Allodynia (variable border)
  - Multiple painful points (Figure 13.1)
  - Nonorganic back signs
  - Incongruent affect
- ○ Normal laboratory studies
- ○ Failure of all prior therapies
- Once an amplified musculoskeletal pain is recognized
  - ○ Acknowledge the pain and explain that it is amplified, not indicative of underlying damage or disease
  - ○ Stop further medical investigations
  - ○ Stop medications
- Restore function
  - ○ Aerobic exercise, up to 5 hours daily of intense therapy focused on functional activities that may take 2 to 3 weeks
  - ○ If allodynia is present, desensitize with tactile stimulation
  - ○ Resume full school attendance
  - ○ Resume social and recreational activities
- Have the psychological dynamics evaluated and appropriately treated
- Anticipate total resolution of symptoms, not just coping or control

References

1. Malleson PN, al-Matar M, Petty RE. Idiopathic musculoskeletal pain syndromes in children. *J Rheumatol*. 1992;19:1786–1789.
2. Merskey DM, Bogduk N. Classification of Chronic Pain. Descriptions of Chronic Pain Syndromes and Definitions of Pain Terms. Seattle: IASP Press, 1994.
3. Wolfe F, Smythe HA, Yunus MB et al. The American College of Rheumatology 1990 Criteria for the Classification of Fibromyalgia. Report of the Multicenter Criteria Committee. *Arthritis Rheum*. 1990;33:160–172.
4. Yunus MB, Masi AT. Juvenile primary fibromyalgia syndrome. A clinical study of thirty-three patients and matched normal controls. *Arthritis Rheum*. 1985;28:138–145.
5. Bowyer S, Roettcher P. Pediatric rheumatology clinic populations in the United States: results of a 3 year survey. Pediatric Rheumatology Database Research Group. *J Rheumatol*. 1996;23:1968–1974.
6. Malleson PN, Fung MY, Rosenberg AM. The incidence of pediatric rheumatic diseases: results from the Canadian Pediatric Rheu-

matology Association Disease Registry. *J Rheumatol.* 1996;23:1981–1987.

7. Manners PJ. Epidemiology of the rheumatic diseases of childhood. *Curr Rheumatol Rep.* 2003;5:453–457.

8. Sherry DD. Pain Syndromes, in Adolescent Rheumatology. In: Isenberg DA, Miller JJI, eds. London: Martin Dunitz Ltd, 1998;197–227.

9. Okifuji A, Turk DC, Sinclair JD et al. A standardized manual tender point survey. I. Development and determination of a threshold point for the identification of positive tender points in fibromyalgia syndrome. *J Rheumatol.* 1997;24:377–383.

10. Rusy LM, Harvey SA, Beste DJ. Pediatric fibromyalgia and dizziness: evaluation of vestibular function. *J Dev Behav Pediatr.* 1999;20:211–215.

11. Laxer RM, Allen RC, Malleson PN et al. Technetium 99m-methylene diphosphonate bone scans in children with reflex neurovascular dystrophy. *J Pediatr.* 1985;106:437–440.

12. Sherry DD. An overview of amplified musculoskeletal pain syndromes. *J Rheumatol.* 2000;58:44–48.

13. Sherry DD, McGuire T, Mellins E et al. Psychosomatic musculoskeletal pain in childhood: clinical and psychological analyses of 100 children. *Pediatrics.* 1991;88:1093–1099.

14. Sherry DD, Wallace CA, Kelley C et al. Short- and long-term outcomes of children with complex regional pain syndrome type I treated with exercise therapy. *Clin J Pain.* 1999;15:218–223.

15. Sherry DD, Weisman R. Psychologic aspects of childhood reflex neurovascular dystrophy. *Pediatrics.* 1988;81:572–578.

16. Sherry DD, Malleson PN. The idiopathic musculoskeletal pain syndromes in childhood. *Rheum Dis Clin North Am.* 2002;28:669–685.

17. Wilder RT, Berde CB, Woldhan M et al. Reflex sympathetic dystrophy in children. Clinical characteristics and follow-up of seventy patients. *J Bone Joint Surg Am.* 1992;74:910–919.

18. Siegel DM, Janeway D, Baum J. Fibromyalgia syndrome in children and adolescents: clinical features at presentation and status at follow-up. *Pediatrics.* 1998;101:377–382.

19. Buskila D, Neumann L, Hershman E et al. Fibromyalgia syndrome in children—an outcome study. *J Rheumatol.* 1995;22:525–528.

20. Walco GA, Ilowite NT. Cognitive-behavioral intervention for juvenile primary fibromyalgia syndrome. *J Rheumatol.* 1992;19:1617–1619.

Chapter 14
Hereditary Conditions of Bone and Cartilage

14.1 INTRODUCTION

Generalized genetic disorders of bone and cartilage growth and development are called skeletal dysplasias or osteochondrodysplasias.[1-3] The International Nosology and Classification of Constitutional Disorders of Bone (2001) identifies about 265 dysplasias, which have been divided into 33 groups, classified according to gene mutations or common patterns of radiological appearances. (Table 14.1). Also included in the classification are the dysostoses, because there is often clinical overlap with the skeletal dysplasias, which leads to diagnostic confusion. The classification identifies three major groups of dysostoses, those with predominant facial and cranial disorders, those with predominant axial involvement, and those with predominant involvement of the extremities.

14.2 EPIDEMIOLOGY

The overall group has a prevalence of between 250 and 350 per million in the population.

14.3 CLINICAL FEATURES

There is often a family history of musculoskeletal problems. Clinical signs include short stature, malformation/shortening of limbs, or dysmorphic features. Often the presentation is one of restriction of movements rather than pain. Pain and stiffness can affect joints as well as the spine. There is no evidence of inflammation. A skeletal survey shows the characteristic abnormalities in the epiphyses and in some, the metaphyses (Figures 14.1 to 14.3). In the dysostosis group, additional clues include the texture of the skin, especially the palms, tendon thickening and shortening (Figure 14.4), a family history of premature osteoarthritis, frequently requiring joint replacement and consanguinity within the family (for autosomal recessive disorders). It is important to search for clinical manifestations in tissues and

TABLE 14.1. Table from the International Nomenclature Classification Including Conditions that May Be Present with Joint Problems

Group Number	Group Heading	Diagnoses
2	Type II collagenopathies	Spondyloepiphyseal dysplasia (SED) Congenital Spondyloepimetaphyseal dysplasia (SEMD) Strudwick type Kniest dysplasia SED Namaqualand type Spondyloperipheral dysplasia Mild SED with premature onset Arthrosis Stickler syndrome type I
3	Type XI collagenopathies	Stickler syndrome type II Marshall syndrome Otospondylomegaepiphyseal dysplasia (OSMED)
11	Other spondyloepi-(meta)-physeal [SE(M)D] dysplasias	X-linked SED tarda SEMD Handigodu type Progressive pseudorheumatoid dysplasia Dyggve–Melchior–Clausen dysplasia Wolcott–Rallison dysplasia Immuno-osseous dysplasia (Schimke) SEMD with joint laxity (SEMDJL) SEMD with multiple dislocations (Hall) SEMD Matillin Type SPONASTRIME dysplasia SEMD short limb-abnormal Calcification type Anauxetic dysplasia

TABLE 14.1. *Continued*

Group Number	Group Heading	Diagnoses
8	Multiple epiphyseal dysplasia and pseudoachondroplasia	Pseudoachondroplasia Multiple epiphyseal dysplasia (MED) Familial hip dysplasia (Beukes)
10	Spondylometaphyseal dysplasias	Spondylometaphyseal dysplasia (SMD) Koslowski type SMD Sutcliffe/corner fracture type SMD with severe genu valgum
13	Brachyolmia spondylodysplasias	Hobaek type Maroteaux type Autosomal dominant type
19	Multiple dislocations with dysplasias	Larsen-like syndromes
26	Dysostosis multiplex group	Mucopolysaccharidosis (MPS) IH MPS IS MPS II MPS IIIA MPS IIIB MPS IIIC MPS IIID MPS IVA MPS IVB MPS VI MPS VII Fucosidosis a-Mannosidosis b-Mannosidosis Aspartylglucosaminuria GM1 gangliosidosis Sialidosis Sialic acid storage disease Galactosialidosis Multiple sulfatase deficiency Mucolipidosis II Mucolipidosis III

TABLE 14.1. *Continued*

Group Number	Group Heading	Diagnoses
27	Osteolyses	Multicentric carpal–tarsal osteolysis with and without nephropathy Winchester syndrome Torg syndrome Hadju–Cheney syndrome Mandibuloacral syndrome Familial expansile osteolysis Juvenile hyaline fibromatosis (including systemic juvenile hyalinosis)

In addition, there are many other disorders involving mutations of collagen that are not a major part of articular cartilage or other structural proteins that can present to the primary-care physician with musculoskeletal complaints. The more common ones are listed below.

Abnormal Protein/Defect	Disorder	Key Features
Type I Collagen	Osteogenesis imperfecta	Fractures, short stature, blue sclerae, dentinogenesis imperfecta
	Idiopathic Juvenile Ostcoporosis	Lower extremity metaphyseal fractures, vertebral fractures, appears around puberty and resolves spontaneously
Types I, III, and V Collagen	Ehlers Danlos syndromes	Manifestations and severity depend on the protein that is abnormal, and include joint hypermobility, skin laxity, doughy skin, nodules, mitral valve prolapse
Fibrillin Type I	Marfan syndrome	Joint hypermobility, tall stature, lens dislocations, high-arched palate, pectus excavatum, aortic root defects
Lubricin	Camptodactyly-arthropathy-coxa vara-pericarditis	Early onset flexion contractures of fingers and toes, progressive noninflammatory polyarthropathy, some patients have pericarditis, others have coxa vara
Cystathionine Synthetase	Homocystinuria Type I	Joint contractures, tall stature, ocular abnormalities, hypotonia, mental retardation

Adapted from references 4 and 5.

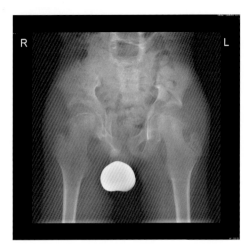

FIGURE 14.1. Pelvic X-ray of a child with Sticklers, showing hypoplasia of iliac wings, thickened femoral neck, metaphyseal irregularities, flattening of femoral epiphysis, acetabular protrusio, and narrowed sciatic notch.

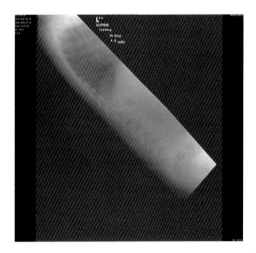

FIGURE 14.2. Spine X-ray of a child with Multiple Epiphyseal Dysplasia, showing abnormal flattened vertebrae: He has a mutation in the matrillin-3 gene.

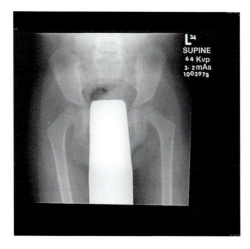

FIGURE 14.3. Pelvic X-ray of a child with Multiple Epiphyseal Dysplasia with mutation in the matrillin-3 gene.

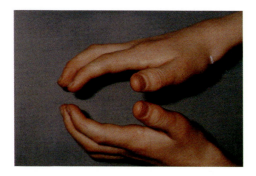

FIGURE 14.4. Hands of a child with mucolipidosis type III: Note the thickened tendons and inability to straighten the fingers.

organs that have the same proteins as the bones and joints as they may help establish a diagnosis (e.g., type II collagen abnormalities also involve the eye and ear; Type XI collagen abnormalities involve the ear but not the eye). Additional examples of patients with mutations of structural proteins are shown in Figures 14.5 to 14.7.

14.4 DIAGNOSIS
A skeletal survey should be obtained on presentation and before the closure of the epiphyses. A diagnosis may be made following identification of the major areas of bone abnormality,

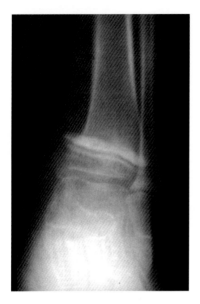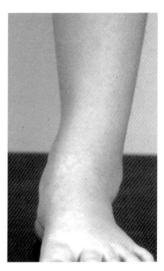

FIGURE 14.5. Clinical photograph and X-ray of a 10-year-old girl who presented with bilateral foot pain and malalignment: The AP view of the left ankle shows subphyseal metaphyseal sclerosis and ankle tilt consistent with metaphyseal fractures typical of idiopathic juvenile osteoporosis.

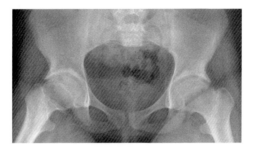

FIGURE 14.6. Frogleg view of the pelvis of a 14-year-old boy with CACP, showing extensive deformity of the hips with mushroom-shaped femoral heads, rounded proximal femoral physes, and acetabular dysplasia.

dislocations, overgrowth, pseudarthroses, short ribs, and club feet. The final diagnosis will include a combination of findings and the name often incorporates the major areas affected—for example, 'craniodiaphyseal dysplasia', 'spondyloepiphyseal

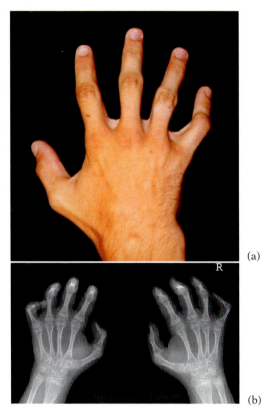

(a)

(b)

FIGURE 14.7. (a) Photograph of the right hand and (b) bilateral hand X-rays of a 14-year-old boy with CACP, showing (a) muscle wasting of the hand and contractures of the PIP joints, and (b) bilateral contractures of multiple digits with enlargement and mild flattening of the metacarpal epiphyses.

dysplasia', or 'acromesomelic dysplasia'. Recent advances in molecular genetics allow for genetic diagnoses to be made in many of these disorders.

14.5 TREATMENT
In the case of dyplasias, maintenance of function with physiotherapy and regular appropriate exercises are all that is necessary. Occasionally pain relief medication will be necessary.

14

In the case of dysostosis multiplex, supportive measures have been the only treatment option for the past decades. Specific enzyme/gene replacement therapies early in the presentation are experimental and promising.

In the idiopathic osteolysis, bisphosphonates have been anecdotally helpful in retarding the progressive osteolysis, but the renal impairment is not responsive.

14.6 PROGNOSIS

Accurate diagnosis of the gene defects are critical to predict the course of the condition. The dysplasias vary in severity and therefore in the functional outcome, but there is usually no compromise to survival. The dysostoses multiplex group from storage diseases are different. They are prone to avascular necrosis in weight bearing joints, and metabolic disease. In the case of osteolysis, the more common one of acro-osteolysis is often associated with renal impairment, as well as progressive functional impairment due to loss of wrist and ankle bones and shortening of phalanges (Figures 14.4, 14.5, and 14.7).

References

1. Hall CM, Washbrook J. *Radiological Electronic Atlas of Malformation Syndromes and Skeletal Dysplasias*. Oxford, UK: Oxford University Press; 2000.
2. Faivre L, Prieur AM, Le Merrer M, Hayem F, Penet C, Woo P et al. Clinical variability and genetic homogeneity of the camptodactyly-arthropathy-coxa vara-pericarditis syndrome. *Am J Med Genet.* 2000; 95:233–236.
3. Norman ME. Juvenile Osteoporosis. In *Primer on the Metabolic Bone Diseases and Disorders of Mineral Metabolism*, Fifth Edition. Favus MJ, ed. Washington, DC: American Society for Bone and Mineral Research, 2003;382–386.
4. Hall C, Woo P. Diseases of Bone and Cartilage in Children. In *Oxford Textbook of Rheumatology*, Third Edition. Isenberg DA, Maddison PJ, Woo P et al, eds. Oxford, UK: Oxford Unviersity Press, 2004;1164–1173.
5. Superti-Furga A, Unger S. Nosology and classification of genetic skeletal disorders, 2006 revision. *Am J Med Genet.* 2006; in Press-Epub.

Index

ACE inhibitors, 81, 84t
Achille's tendon, 40f
Acute rheumatic fever (ARF),
   137–140
  cardiac symptoms in, 138
  diagnosis/differential diagnosis
   in, 138–139
  epidemiology and etiology of,
   137
  treatment and outcomes of,
   139
Alkaline phosphatase, 9
Allodynia, 158–159, 162
Alveolitis, inflammatory, 81–82,
  84t
Amoxicillin, 120, 121t
Amplified musculoskeletal pain,
  155–164
  definition of, 155
  diagnosis and treatment in,
   159–164
  epidemiology of, 157
  etiology and clinical
   manifestations in, 158–159
  outcome and key points in,
   162–164
  working model of, 161f
Amyloidosis, familial, 128–129,
  132, 133
Anakinra, 133, 134, 135
ANCA (antineutrophil
  cytoplasmic antibodies),
  110–112
Anemias, 56

Aneurysms
  of coronary arteries, 102–104
  in polyarteritis nodosa/
   necrotizing vasculitis, 106,
   107f
  of pulmonary arteries, 115–116
Angiography (Kawasaki disease),
  104f
Ankle joints, 25f
Ankylosing spondylitis (AS), 41,
  42t, 160
Antibiotics, 120, 121t, 139–140
Antibodies
  in Lyme disease, 119–120
  in mixed connective tissue
   disease, 92
  myositis-specific, 67t, 73
  in systemic lupus
   erythematosus, 50t, 56–58,
   62, 64
Antidepressants, 160–161
Antimyeloperoxidase (anti-MPO),
  111
Antineutrophil cytoplasmic
  antibodies (ANCA),
  110–112
Antinuclear antibody (ANA) test
  cautions about, 9
  iridocyclitis and, 25–26, 27t
  in juvenile dermatomyositis, 73
  in mixed connective tissue
   disease, 90, 92
  in Raynaud's phenomenon, 79
  in sclerodermas, 83, 85t

Page numbers followed by f indicate figures; t, tables.

Antinuclear antibody (ANA) test
    (*cont.*)
    in Sjögren's syndrome, 95
    speckled pattern in, 91–92
    in systemic lupus
        erythematosus, 50t, 56–57
Antiphospholipid antibody
    syndrome (APLS), 53, 55
Anti-sIL-6R, 17
Antistreptolysin O (ASO) titre,
    138
Anti-TNF agents
    action of, 17
    for Behçet's disease, 115t
    for juvenile idiopathic arthritis,
        29t, 30, 32t
    for polyarteritis nodosa/
        necrotizing vasculitis, 108,
        112
Arteritis, *see* Vasculitis
Arthritis; *see also specific diseases*
    as differential diagnosis, 160
    episodic, 13t
    Lyme arthritis, *see* Lyme disease
    migratory, 13t, 138
    in mixed connective tissue
        disease, 92
    monoarticular, 12t
    nonmigratory, 140–141
Aspirin, 104
Autoantibody production, 47,
    73
Autoimmune thrombocytopenic
    purpura (AITP), 55–56
Autoinflammatory syndromes,
    123–136; *see also* Fevers,
    recurrent/syndromal;
    specific syndromes
    chronic infantile neurological
        cutaneous and articular
        syndrome (CINCA),
        124–127, 134–135
    CIAS 1 syndromes, 124–127,
        133
    as differential diagnosis, 135
    familial cold autoinflammatory
        syndrome (FCAS), 124–127,
        133, 134t

familial Mediterranean fever
    (FMF), 123–129
hyperimmunoglobulinemia D
    syndrome (HIDS), 124–127,
    129–131
information tables on,
    124–127
key points in, 135–136
Muckle–Well syndrome (MWS),
    124–127, 133–134
periodic fever, aphthous
    stomatitis, pharyngitis and
    adenopathy syndrome,
    124–127, 129
prevalence/incidence of, 14t
tumor necrosis factor-receptor-
    associated periodic
    syndrome (TRAPS),
    124–127, 131–133
Azathioprine
    action of, 17–18
    for Behçet's disease, 115t
    for polyarteritis nodosa/
        necrotizing vasculitis,
        108
    for systemic lupus
        erythematosus, 59–60

Back pain, 5
Behçet's disease (BD), 113–116
    diagnostic criteria for, 114
    ethnicity and, 113–114
    pharmacologic management of,
        17
    treatment algorithm for, 115t
Beighton Scale of Hypermobility,
    146t
Bell's palsy, 118–121
Benign hypermobility syndrome
    (BHMS), 145–150
    physical exam for, 146–149
Biopsies
    renal, 110
    of skin, 100, 110
Bisphosphonates, 174
Bohan and Peter Diagnostic
    Criteria (for JDM), 67t

Bones, *see* Musculoskeletal disorders; *specific bones*
Borrelia burgdorferi spirochete, 118
Brain
increased intracranial pressure in, 135
MRI of, 71f

Calcaneous, 151
Calcinosis, 69, 75, 80f
Camptodactyly-arthropathy-coxa vara pericarditis (CACP), 169f, 172f, 173f
Cardiac disorders
camptodactyly-arthropathy-coxa vara pericarditis (CACP), 169t, 172f, 173f
in Kawasaki disease, 102–104
in Lyme disease, 118–119, 121
in sclerodermas, 82
in systemic lupus erythematosus, 56, 62, 64
Carpal joints, 147t
Cefuroxime axetil, 120, 121t
Central nervous system
in Behçet's disease, 114, 116
in juvenile dermatomyositis, 70
in Lyme disease, 121t
Cervical spine
examination of, 6
juvenile idiopathic arthritis in, 24
Chorea (St. Vitus' dance), 138
Chronic infantile neurologic cutaneous and articular syndrome (CINCA), 124–127, 134–135
arthropathy/ossification in, 134–135
as differential diagnosis, 37t, 101
symptoms table for, 125–127
CIAS 1 gene, 133
CIAS 1 syndromes, 124–127, 133
symptoms table for, 125–127

CINCA, *see* Chronic infantile neurologic cutaneous and articular syndrome (CINCA)
Clubbing, 12t, 172
Cognitive behavior therapy, 163
Colchicine
action of, 17–18
for Behçet's disease, 115
for familial Mediterranean fever, 128–129
for polyarteritis nodosa/ necrotizing vasculitis, 108
Cold exposure, 133, 134
Collagenopathies, 167t
Complementary and alternative therapies, 19, 162
Complex regional pain syndrome type 1 (CRPS1), 155, 158–162
Computerized tomography (CT) scans
of temporomandibular joint (TMJ), 6f
of upper respiratory tract, 112, 113f
Congenital heart block (CHB), 62, 64
Connective tissue diseases (CTDs)
as differential diagnosis, 58t
list of classic, 90
Contractures
in juvenile dermatomyositis, 68
in PIP joints, 173f
Control point testing, 158–159
Coombs' positive hemolytic anemia, 56–57
Coronary artery aneurysms, 102–104
Costochondritis, 151
Creatine kinase (CK), 72, 75
Cryopyrin, 133
CT, *see* Computerized tomography (CT) scans
Cutaneous polyarteritis, 108–110
CVA, *see* Stroke (cerebrovascular accident)

Cyanosis, 158–159
Cyclophosphamide
   action of, 17–18
   for Behçet's disease, 115t
   for juvenile dermatomyositis, 74t, 75
   for polyarteritis nodosa/ necrotizing vasculitis, 108
   for sclerodermas, 84t
   for systemic lupus erythematosus, 59–60
Cyclosporine
   action of, 17–18
   for Behçet's disease, 115t
   for juvenile dermatomyositis, 74t
   for systemic lupus erythematosus, 59–60
Cytokines, 17–19

Dactylitis
   differential diagnosis for, 12t
   in psoriatic arthritis, 44t
Deafness, sensorineural, 134, 135
D8/17 cell surface marker, 137
Deoxyribonuclease B (anti-Dnase B), 138–139
Depression
   in amplified musculoskeletal pain, 160–161
   in systemic lupus erythematosus, 53
Diclofenac, 42
Discoid rash, 49t, 51–52
Doxycycline, 120, 121t
Drugs; *see also specific drugs*
   ACE inhibitors, 81, 84t
   antibiotics, 120, 121t, 139–140
   antidepressants, 160–161
   anti-TNF agents, 17, 29t, 30, 32t, 108, 112, 115t
   bisphosphonates, 174
   for cell targeting, 17–18
   lupus-inducing, 64
   prophylactic, 109–110, 139–140

   for soluble mediator targeting, 17
   vasodilators, 84t
Dry eyes and mouth
   in Sjögren's syndrome, 94f
   in systemic lupus erythematosus, 51–52
Dysostoses, 166, 168t, 174
Dysphagia, 75, 80–81, 94
Dysphonia, 69
Dysplasias, skeletal, 166–174
   clinical manifestations of, 166, 170t
   diagnosis/differential diagnosis in, 171–173
   grouping tables for, 167–169
   treatment and outcomes in, 173–174

Edema
   of hands, 79, 90, 91f
   of soft tissue, 68
Ehlers–Danlos syndrome, 147, 149
Elbow joints
   examination of, 6, 7t
   pain in, 152
Electromyelography, 67t
En coup de sabre lesions, 86–87
Endocarditis
   in acute rheumatic fever, 138–140
   in systemic lupus erythematosus, 56
Entheses
   most commonly involved, 7–8
   of tibial tubercle, 150–151
Enthesitis, 11t
Enthesitis-related arthritis (ERA), 39–43
   defined, 39
   diagnosis/differential diagnosis in, 40–41, 42t
   epidemiology, etiology, and manifestations of, 39
   treatment and outcomes in, 42–43

Enzymes
serum muscle enzymes, 67t, 72, 75
in streptococcal antigens, 139
Epicondylitis, 152
Erysipelas-like skin lesions, 124, 128f
Erythema marginatum, 130f, 138
Erythema migrans, 119f, 121t
Erythrocyte sedimentation rate (ESR), 9, 57, 82
Erythromycin, 139t
Etanercept
for hyperimmunoglobulinemia D syndrome, 131
for TRAPS, 133
Ethnicity/racial predilection
acute rheumatic fever and, 137
amplified musculoskeletal pain and, 157
Behçet's disease and, 113–114
familial Mediterranean fever and, 128
prevalence/incidence by, 14t
systemic lupus erythematosus and, 47
TRAPS and, 131
European Spondyloarthropathy Study Group (ESSG) criteria, 41, 42t
Exercise therapy, *see* Physiotherapy/physical therapy

Familial cold autoinflammatory syndrome (FCAS), 124–137, 133, 134t
symptoms table for, 125–127
Familial hibernian fever, *see* Tumor necrosis factor-receptor-associated periodic syndrome (TRAPS)
Familial Mediterranean fever (FMF), 123–129
diagnosis, treatment, and outcomes in, 128–129

epidemiology, etiology, and manifestations of, 123–128
genetic component in, 123–124
symptoms table for, 125–127
Family history, 3–5, 166
Femoral head, 152–153
Fevers
in Kawasaki disease, 102
recurrent/syndromal, 123–136
in systemic juvenile idiopathic arthritis, 35f
Fractures
of femoral head, 153
microavulsion, 150–151

Gabapentin, 161
Gammaglobulin, intravenous, 104
Gastrointestinal disorders
in Behçet's disease, 114, 116
gastroprotection for, 73–74
in hyperimmunoglobulinemia D syndrome, 130
in juvenile dermatomyositis, 69–70
in sclerodermas, 80–81, 84t, 85t
in systemic lupus erythematosus, 56
Gender/sex predilection
amplified musculoskeletal pain and, 157
prevalence/incidence by, 14t
Genetics/genes
CIAS 1 syndromes and, 133
familial Mediterranean fever (FMF) and, 123–124, 128
hereditary conditions of bone and cartilage, 166–174
HLA-B27, 26, 28t, 39
HLADR3 phenotypes, 94
hyperimmunoglobulinemia D syndrome (HIDS) and, 129–131
M694V genotype, 128
psoriatic arthritis and, 43–44
systemic juvenile idiopathic arthritis and, 34–35

Genetics/genes (*cont.*)
    testing for, 136
    TRAPS and, 131–133
Genital ulcers, 114
Glomerulonephritis, 110
Glucocorticoids, *see* Steroids
Gottron's papules, 68
Group A β hemolytic streptococci, 137
"Growing pains," 150

Hand joints, 31, 33
Hands
    edema of, 79, 90, 91f
    with mucolipidosis, 171f
    rash on palms, 130
    rhythmic squeezing of, 138
Headache
    in CINCA syndrome, 135
    in systemic lupus erythematosus, 53
Heart, *see* Cardiac disorders
Heel pain, 151
Heliotrope rash, 68, 94f
Hematologic disorders
    in sclerodermas, 83
    in systemic lupus erythematosus, 50t, 55–61
Henoch–Schönlein purpura (HSP), 97–100
    classification criteria for, 98t
Hepatitis B-associated PAN, 106, 108
Hepatomegaly, 130
Hereditary conditions of bone and cartilage, 166–174
    clinical manifestations of, 166, 170t
    diagnosis/differential diagnosis in, 171–173
    grouping tables for, 167–169
    treatment and outcomes in, 173–174
Hip joints
    fractures of, 153
    hypermobility of, 148–149
    idiopathic chondrolysis of, 154

pain in, 11t, 152
    septic hip, 152
Histocompatibility locus antigen (HLA), 26, 28t, 39, 93, 114
HLA-B27 test, 26, 28t, 39, 140
HLA-B51 test, 114
HLADR3 phenotypes, 94
Homeopathy, 19
Hydroxychloroquine
    action of, 17–18
    for systemic lupus erythematosus, 59–61
Hyperimmunoglobulinemia D syndrome (HIDS), 124–127, 129–131
    diagnosis, treatment, and outcomes in, 130–131
    epidemiology, etiology, and manifestations of, 129–130
    genetic component in, 129–131
    symptoms table for, 125–127
Hypermobility, joint, 145–150
Hypocomplementemia, 57
Hypocomplementemic urticarial vasculitis, 101
Hypothyroidism, 153

Idiopathic chondrolysis of hip, 154
Idiopathic juvenile osteoporosis, 169t, 172f
IgA, *see* Immunoglobulin serum antibodies
IL-1ra, 17
Imaging studies; *see also specific tests*
    for mechanical/orthopedic conditions, 154
    of temporomandibular joint (TMJ), 6f
Immune system; *see also specific immune disorders*
    dysregulation symptoms in, 23
    in systemic lupus erythematosus, 47, 50t, 55–56

Immunoglobulin serum
antibodies
A (IgA), 99
D (IgD), 129–130
I (IgG), 119–120
M (IgM), 119–120
Increased intracranial pressure
(ICCP), 135
Indomethacin, 36, 42
Infection
as differential diagnosis, 37t,
58t
systemic viral, 58t
upper respiratory, 102,
107f
Inflammation
of airway, 112
characteristics of, 3
glandular, 94
of joints, *see specific joints*
of muscles, *see* Muscles/
myalgias
of tendons and ligaments, *see*
Enthesitis-related arthritis
(ERA)
Inflammatory rheumatologic
diseases
acute rheumatic fever,
137–140
characteristics of, 3–5
juvenile dermatomyositis/
polymyositis, 66–75
juvenile idiopathic arthritis,
23–45
overlap syndromes in, 90–95
pharmacologic management of,
16–18
post streptococcal reactive
arthritis, 140–141
recurrent/syndromal,
123–136
sclerodermas, 77–88
systemic lupus erythematosus,
47–64
vasculitis, 97–116
Infliximab, 108, 112
Injections, intra-articular, 30
Interstitial cystitis (IC), 56

Interstitial lung fibrosis, 81–83,
84t, 85t, 92
Iridocyclitis (uveitis)
in Behçet's disease, 114–116
in CINCA syndrome, 135
in juvenile idiopathic arthritis,
24–26
Ixodes ticks, 118

Jaw, *see* Temporomandibular
joint (TMJ) excursion
Joints; *see also specific joints and
diseases*
contractures of, 68
examination of, 6–8
hypermobility of, 145–150
injection of, 30
ossification in, 134
pelvic, 173f
Juvenile dermatomyositis/
polymyositis, 66–75
with associated rheumatologic
disease, 70
characteristics of, 18–19
classical, 68–69
diagnosis/differential diagnosis
in, 67t, 72–73
overview of, 66–67
prevalence/incidence of,
14t
prognosis/outcome in, 75
sine myositis, 69, 70f
treatment of, 73–75
with vasculopathy, 70
Juvenile idiopathic arthritis (JIA),
23–45
as differential diagnosis, 58t
enthesitis-related (ERA),
39–43
oligoarthritis, 23–30
overview of, 23, 24t
polyarthritis, rheumatoid factor
negative, 31–33
prevalence/incidence of, 14t
psoriatic, 28–29, 43–44
systematic (sJIA), 34–38
unclassified, 45

Kawasaki disease (KD), 101–105
classification criteria for, 102t
as differential diagnosis, 37t
laboratory evaluations in,
103–104
treatment of, 104–105
Keratoconjunctivitis sicca
in Sjögren's syndrome, 94–95
in systemic lupus
erythematosus, 51–52
Kidneys, see Renal disorders
Knee joints
hypermobility of, 148–149
juvenile idiopathic arthritis in,
24
Lyme arthritis in, 119–120
microavulsion fractures of,
150–151
pain in, 11t

Laboratory evaluations
in acute rheumatic fever,
138–139
in Henoch–Schölein purpura,
99
in hypocomplementemic
urticarial vasculitis, 101
in Kawasaki disease, 103–104
in Lyme disease, 119–120
for mechanical/orthopedic
conditions, 154
in sclerodermas, 82–83
of serum muscle enzymes, 67t
in Sjögren's syndrome, 95
in Wegener's granulomatosis,
112
Leflunamide, 17–18
Legg–Calvé–Perthes disease,
152–153
Leukemia (as differential
diagnosis), 37t
Leukocytoclastic/hypersensitivity
vasculitis, 100–101
Ligaments, see Tendons and
ligaments
Linear scleroderma, 86–87
Livedo rashes, 106f

Lower back examination, 6–7, 8f
Lupus nephritis, 49t, 53–55, 54t
Lyme disease, 118–121
clinical manifestations and
diagnosis of, 119–120
prevalence/incidence of, 14t, 118
treatment and outcomes in,
120–121

Macular rash, 62, 63f
Magnetic resonance imaging
(MRI), 71f
Malar rash, 49t, 51–52, 62, 63f
Malignancies (as differential
diagnoses), 37t, 58t, 95, 160
Marfan syndrome, 149
Mechanical/orthopedic
conditions, 145–154
benign hypermobility
syndrome, 145–150
Osgood–Schlatter syndrome,
150–151
other various, 151–154
physical exam for, 146–149
MEFV gene, 123–124
Meningitis, 135
Metacarpal joints, 31, 33, 146t
Methotrexate
action of, 17
for juvenile dermatomyositis,
74t
for juvenile idiopathic arthritis,
29t, 30, 32t
for sclerodermas, 88
for systemic lupus
erythematosus, 60t
for Wegener's granulomatosis,
113
Methylprednisolone
for Behçet's disease, 115t
for cutaneous polyarteritis, 110
for juvenile dermatomyositis,
73–75
for Kawasaki disease, 104
for polyarteritis
nodosa/necrotizing
vasculitis, 108

for systemic lupus
erythematosus, 59
Mevalonate kinase (MVK),
129–131
Microavulsion fractures, 150–151
Microscopic polyangiitis, 110–111
Mitral valve, 138–140
Mixed connective tissue disease
(MCTD), 90–94
diagnosis/differential diagnosis
in, 92
outcomes for, 92–93
overview of, 90–92
treatment of, 93
Monoclonal antibodies to B cells,
17–18
M694V genotype, 128
Muckle–Well syndrome (MWS),
124–127, 133–134
symptoms table for, 125–127
Mucolipidosis, 168t, 171f
Mucus membranes
in Behçet's disease, 114
in Sjögren's syndrome, 94–95
in systemic lupus
erythematosus, 51–52
Multiple epiphyseal dysplasia
(MED), 168t, 170f, 171f
Muscles/myalgias
biopsy abnormalities in, 67t,
72–73
fibromyalgia, 155–157
in juvenile dermatomyositis,
71f
in mixed connective tissue
disease, 92
in polymyositis, 71–72
serum enzymes of, 67t, 72,
75
in TRAPS, 132
weakness of, 67–69
Musculoskeletal disorders
amplified pain in, 155–164
in dermatomyositis/
polymyositis, 70–73
mechanical/orthopedic
conditions, 145–154
in sclerodermas, 80

Mycophenolate mofetil, 17–18
Myeloperoxidase (MPO), 110–112
Myocarditis
in acute rheumatic fever,
138–140
in Kawasaki disease, 102–103
in systemic lupus
erythematosus, 56
Myositis, *see* Juvenile
dermatomyositis/
polymyositis

Nail changes, 43–44
Neck, *see* Cervical spine
Necrosis of femoral head,
152–153
Necrotizing vasculitis, 106, 107f,
109
Neonatal lupus erythematosus
(NLE), 62–64
Neonatal onset multisystem
inflammatory disease
(NOMID), 37t
Neuroblastoma, 37t
Neurologic disorders
in CINCA syndrome, 135
differential diagnosis for, 12t
in Lyme disease, 118–119,
121
in systemic lupus
erythematosus, 49t,
53–55
Neutrophilic pleocytosis,
135
NOMID (neonatal onset
multisystem inflammatory
disease), 37t
Noninflammatory rheumatologic
diseases, 145–174
mechanical/orthopedic
conditions, 145–154
benign hypermobility
syndrome (BHMS),
145–150
Osgood–Schlatter syndrome,
150–151
other various, 151–154

Nonsteroidal anti-inflammatory drugs (NSAIDs)
action of, 17
for enthesitis, 42
for juvenile idiopathic arthritis, 29t, 30, 32t

Observation hip, 152
Oligoarthritis
clinical manifestations of, 24–26
defined, 23
diagnosis/differential diagnosis in, 26, 28t
epidemiology and etiology of, 24
treatment and outcomes in, 29t, 30
Oral ulcers, 49t, 51–52, 114, 129
Osgood–Schlatter syndrome, 150–151
Ossification, 134
Osteolyses, 169t
Osteonecrosis, 151
Osteopenia/osteoporosis
idiopathic juvenile, 169f, 172f
steroids and, 52
Overlap syndromes, 90–95
mixed connective tissue disease, 90–94
Sjögren's syndrome, 94–95

Pain
amplified musculoskeletal, 155–164
in back, see Back pain
in bones/skeletal system, 13t
characteristics of, 4t, 18
in elbow, 152
in heel, 151
in hip joints, 11t, 152
behind knees, 11t
in mechanical/orthopedic conditions, 145, 150
monoarticular, 12t
syndrome prevalence of, 14t

Parotid glands, 94f
Parry–Romberg syndrome, 86–88
Pathergy phenomenon, 114
Penicillin, prophylactic, 109–110, 139–140
Pericarditis
in acute rheumatic fever, 138–140
camptodactyly-arthropathy-coxa vara pericarditis, 169t, 172f, 173f
in Kawasaki disease, 102–103
in Lyme disease, 121t
in sclerodermas, 82
in systemic lupus erythematosus, 49t, 53
Perinuclear antineutrophil cytoplasmic antibodies (p-ANCA), 110
Periodic fever, aphthous stomatitis, pharyngitis and adenopathy (PFAPA) syndrome, 124–127, 129
symptoms table for, 125–127
Peripheral vasculitis, 51–52
Peritonitis
in familial Mediterranean fever, 124
in systemic lupus erythematosus, 56
Phalangeal joints, 31, 33
Photosensitivity, 49t, 59–60, 94
Physiotherapy/physical therapy
for amplified musculoskeletal pain, 162–164
for dysplasias, 173
for juvenile dermatomyositis, 75
Pilocarpine, 95
Piroxicam, 42
Plantar fasciitis, 40f
Plaque morphea, 85–86
Plasmapheresis, 61t, 108, 111
Pleural effusions, 81–82, 84t
Pleuritis
in familial Mediterranean fever, 124
in sclerodermas, 81–82, 84t

in systemic lupus erythematosus, 49t, 53
Pneumothorax, 110–111
Polyarteritis nodosa (PAN)/necrotizing vasculitis, 105–108
classification criteria for, 105t
hepatitis B-associated, 106, 108
Polyarthritis, rheumatoid factor (RF) negative, 31–33
Polyarthritis, rheumatoid factor (RF) positive, 32t, 33–34
Polymyositis, 71–72, 66–75
Post streptococcal reactive arthritis (PSRA), 140–141
Pressure measurements, 134–135
Prophylaxis, 109–110, 139–140
Proteinase 3 (PR3), 111–112
Proteins, abnormal/defective, 169t; see also Genetics/genes
Psoriasis, 43–44
Psoriatic arthritis, 43–44
Psychodynamics, 162
Pulmonary disorders
in Behçet's disease, 115–116
in familial Mediterranean fever, 124
in microscopic polyangiitis, 111
in sclerodermas, 81–82, 84t, 92
in systemic lupus erythematosus, 49t, 53, 56
Pulmonary function tests (PFTs), 82
Pulmonary hypertension, 81–82, 84t, 92
Pyrin (marenostrin), 123, 133

Racial predilection, see Ethnicity/racial predilection
Radiography
of chest, 112–113
joint ossification on, 134
in Legg–Calvé–Perthes disease, 152–153
pelvic, 170–172

Rashes; see also specific rashes
in acute rheumatic fever, 138
in Behçet's disease, 114, 116
in CINCA syndrome, 134–135
conditions associated/not associated with, 72t
in cutaneous polyarteritis, 109
differential diagnosis for, 12t
in Henoch–Schölein purpura, 99f
in hyperimmunoglobulinemia D syndrome, 130
in hypocomplementemic urticarial vasculitis, 101
in juvenile dermatomyositis, 67t, 68
in juvenile idiopathic arthritis, 35f
in leukocytoclastic/hypersensitivity vasculitis, 100
in Lyme disease, 119f, 121t
in neonatal lupus erythematosus, 62, 63f
in polyarteritis nodosa/necrotizing vasculitis, 106f
in systemic lupus erythematosus, 49t, 51–52
in TRAPS, 132
Raynaud's phenomenon
differential diagnosis in, 13t, 78
in mixed connective tissue disease, 90, 92
in scleroderma classification, 85t
treatment of, 84t
Reflex sympathetic dystrophy, see Complex regional pain syndrome type 1 (CRPS1)
Reflux esophagitis, 81, 84t, 85t
Renal disorders
in Henoch–Schölein purpura, 99–100
in microscopic polyangiitis, 111
in mixed connective tissue disease, 92
in sclerodermas, 81

Renal disorders (*cont.*)
  in systemic lupus
    erythematosus, 49t, 53–55,
    54t
Reynaud's phenomenon, 52
Rheumatoid factor (RF)
  in polyarthritis, 31–34
  in Sjögren's syndrome, 95
Rheumatologic diseases
  acute versus chronic, 10t
  differential diagnosis/diagnostic
    clues in, 9, 11–13
  etiology of, 9
  illness patterns in, 10t
  inflammatory/autoimmune, *see*
    Inflammatory
    rheumatologic diseases
  joint examination in, 6–8
  lab and imaging studies in, 6–8;
    see also specific tests
  management principles in,
    16–20
    multidisciplinary, 18–20
    pharmacological, 17–18
  noninflammatory, *see*
    Noninflammatory
    rheumatologic diseases
  overview of, 3–5
  patient history in, 3–5, 166
  physical examination in, 5
  prevalence/incidence in, 14t,
    15
  systemic versus localized, 10t
Rheumatologic fever, acute, 14t
Rheumatologic history patterns,
    3–5, 166
Rider and Targoff Diagnostic
    Criteria (for JDM), 67t
Ro and La antibodies, 56, 62, 64,
    94, 95

Schober test, 7, 8f
Sclerodactyly, 84–85
Sclerodermas, 77–88
  characteristics of, 19
  classification criteria for, 84t,
    85t

  clinical manifestations of,
    78–82
  diagnosis/differential diagnosis
    in, 82–83, 84t, 85t
  epidemiology and etiology of,
    77, 78t
  outcomes in, 83
  prevalence/incidence of, 14t
  treatment of, 83, 84t, 85t, 88
Seizures, 53
Septic hip, 152
Serial casting, 30
Serositis, 49t, 53
Sever syndrome, 151
Sex predilection, *see* Gender/sex
    predilection
Shoulder joints, 147t
Shrinking lung syndrome, 56
Sicca syndrome/complex, 56, 93
Sinding–Larsen–Johannson
    syndrome, 151
Sine myositis, 69, 70f
Sjögren's syndrome (SS), 93–95
  diagnosis, treatment, and
    outcomes in, 95
  overview of, 93
  prevalence and disease course
    in, 94
Skin; *see also rashes*
  amplified pain in, 158–159, 162
  biopsy of, 100, 110
  cyanosis of, 158–159
  erysipelas-like lesions on, 124,
    128f
  exceptional elasticity of, 149
  in juvenile dermatomyositis,
    67–70
  in neonatal lupus
    erythematosus, 62, 63f
  in sclerodermas, 83–88, 97
  in systemic lupus
    erythematosus, 49t, 51–52
  ulcers on, 70f
Sleep, 162
Slipped capitol femoral epiphysis
    (SCFE), 153
Slit lamp examination, 27t
Social history, 4–5

Splenomegaly, 130
Spondyloarthropathy, 41, 42t, 160, 167t
Staphylococcus aureus, 152
Stem cell transplants, autologous, 17–18
Steroids
  action of, 17–18
  for Behçet's disease, 115
  for cutaneous polyarteritis, 110
  for Henoch–Schölein purpura, 100
  injection of, 30
  intra-articular, 120
  for juvenile dermatomyositis, 73
  for Kawasaki disease, 104
  for leukocytoclastic/ hypersensitivity vasculitis, 100–101
  osteopenia and, 52
  for systemic lupus erythematosus, 59–61
Stickler dysplasias, 167t, 170f
Streptococcal disease, 137–141
Stroke (cerebrovascular accident), 53
Sulfadiazine, 139t
Sulfasalazine, 17–18
Swallowing difficulty, *see* Dysphagia
Synovitis, 120, 152
Systematic juvenile idiopathic arthritis (sJIA), 34–38
  clinical manifestations of, 35–36
  diagnosis/differential diagnosis in, 36, 37t
  epidemiology and etiology of, 34–35
  outcomes for, 37–38
  treatment of, 36–37, 38t
Systemic lupus erythematosus (SLE), 47–64
  classification criteria for, 48–50
  clinical manifestations of, 48–56
    antiphospholipid antibody syndrome, 55
    hematologic, 55–61
    mucocutaneous, 51–52
    musculoskeletal, 52–53
    neurologic, serosal, renal, 53–55
    other various, 56
  diagnosis/differential diagnosis in, 56–57, 58t
  as differential diagnosis, 37t
  drug-induced, 64
  etiology of, 47–48
  long-term morbidity in, 48t
  neonatal (NLE), 62–64
  prevalence/incidence of, 14t
  prognosis/outcome in, 62
  treatment of, 57, 59–61
Systemic sclerosis (SSc), *see* Sclerodermas

Temporomandibular joint (TMJ) excursion, 6, 7f
Tendons and ligaments
  Achilles tendon, 4f
  attachments to bone, *see* Entheses
  inflammation of, *see* Enthesitis-related arthritis (ERA)
  infrapatellar, 150–151
Tests, *see specific tests*
Thalidomide
  action of, 17–18
  for Behçet's disease, 115
  for systemic lupus erythematosus, 60t
Tibial tubercle, 150–151
Tickborne diseases, 118
Tietze syndrome, 151
TNFRSF1A gene, 131–133
Torticollis, 25
Toxic synovitis, 152
Tramadol, 161
Transient synovitis, 152
TRAPS, *see* Tumor necrosis factor-receptor-associated periodic syndrome (TRAPS)
Triamcinolone hexacetonide, 30

Trigger points, 155–159
Tumor necrosis factor-receptor-associated periodic syndrome (TRAPS), 124–127, 131–133
  chronicity of, 133
  diagnosis, treatment, and outcomes in, 132–133
  epidemiology, etiology, and manifestations of, 131–132
  symptoms table for, 125–127

Ulcers
  genital, 114
  oral, 49t, 51–52, 114, 129
  skin, 70f
U1RNP antibody, 90–91
Upper respiratory tract infections, 102, 107f
Uveitis, *see* Iridocyclitis (uveitis)

Valgus deformity, 25f
Vasculitis, 97–116
  Behçet's disease, 113–116
  in bowel, 56
  cutaneous polyarteritis, 108–110
  as differential diagnosis, 37t, 58t
  Henoch–Schönlein purpura (HSP), 97–100
  hypocomplementemic urticarial vasculitis, 101
  in juvenile dermatomyositis, 70

  Kawasaki disease, 101–105
  leukocytoclastic/hypersensitivity vasculitis, 100–101
  microscopic polyangiitis, 110–111
  necrotizing, 106, 107f, 109
  new classification of childhood vasculitis, 98t
  in polyarteritis nodosa/necrotizing vasculitis, 105–108
  prevalence/incidence of, 14t
  pulmonary, 56, 70
  in sclerodermas, 81–83, 84t
  in systemic lupus erythematosus, 51–52
  Wegener's granulomatosis, 110f, 111–113
Vasodilators, peripheral, 84t
Viral infection, 58t

Wegener's granulomatosis (WG), 110f, 111–113
  chronicity of, 113
  classification criteria for, 111t
Western blot testing, 119–120

Xerostomia, 51–52, 94f

Yunus and Masi criteria for fibromyalgia in children, 156t

Printed in Singapore